SPARROW IN THE HALL

60 years of medical practice in England, Nigeria and Australia

ROBIN JELLIFFE

Nenge Books, Australia

Sparrow in the Hall

by Robin Jelliffe

Copyright © Robin Jelliffe 2008

All rights reserved.

This book is copyright. Except as permitted under the Copyright Act 1968, (for example a fair dealing for the purposes of study, research, criticism or review) no part of this book may be reproduced, stored in a retrieval system, or transmitted in any form or by any means without prior written permission of the publisher.

First edition published in 2008 (ISBN 9781740185615)

Second edition 2021
Published by Nenge Books, Australia
nengebooks1@gmail.com
www.nengebooks.com

All photographs are copyright © Robin Jelliffe except on:
front cover - copyright unknown (untraceable former Advocate photo);
page 247 - copyright © North Coast News

ISBN 978-0-6488889-1-8

CONTENTS

Foreword	5
Introduction	7
Chapter 1: Childhood	13
Chapter 2: Medical Student	41
Chapter 3: Clinical Student	52
Chapter 4: Resident	77
Chapter 5: Out to Africa	88
Chapter 6: Azare	101
Chapter 7: Kano and Kaduna	131
Chapter 8: Ibadan	149
Chapter 9: Nottingham and Shotley Bridge	155
Chapter 10: Out to Australia	163
Chapter 11: Goondiwindi	169
Chapter 12: Family Doctor - 1	184
Chapter 13: Flying	198
Chapter 14: New Guinea Interludes	206
Chapter 15: Family Doctor - 2	221
Chapter 16: Hospital Superintendent	228
Chapter 17: Final Stretch	247
Endnotes	259

FOREWORD

This updated second edition has been published by the author's family due to requests for the book after the first edition became out of print. It comes on the first anniversary of his death on January 11th, 2020, almost 92 years old, and includes some additional photographs which add to the visual impact of his narrative as well as the visual historical record, important for family. Robin left Jill, three surviving sons, eight grandchildren and eight great-grandchildren.

We hope that future readers will be as enthralled by the author's experiences and insights into the 20th century as previous readers have been, recording a time of change, innovation and technological enterprise unrivaled in the history of the planet. This edition, available through print-on-demand publishing, will also enable a wider readership to appreciate the author's extraordinary life and his contribution to the lives of many others, particularly in medicine and health care. For us as family, his story provides a legacy of our own family history, preserved now for the future, including the recognition and appreciation of the life of this man who was much loved.

Michael Jelliffe
January 2021

INTRODUCTION

As if, when you are sitting at dinner with your chiefs and ministers in wintertime, one of the sparrows from outside flew very quickly through the hall; as if it came in one door and went out through another. Man's life appears to be more or less like this; and of what may follow it, or what preceded it, we are absolutely ignorant.

The Venerable Bede, A.D. 731

They slip back into the mists of the past, my ancestral ghosts, the sources of my genetic structure, each one a complete life, yet each one anonymous, each one part of me. Their lives are foreshortened to entries in yearly parish returns, christenings, marriages and burials, preserved on paper and parchment in diocesan records. Hand written in illegible scrawls, equally illegibly precise classical style, or meticulous copperplate, they tell nothing of their hopes and aspirations, passions, crimes and crises. Within their short term on earth, each one felt special and unique. They ate, slept, fell in and out of love, gained and lost wealth, became parents, became old and died. They leave one line in an annual report from a church warden, an old will, a fading sepia-tinted photograph or an inscription on a crumbling tombstone. Ironically, in this age of technology, I am converting my life story into a 12 centimetre diameter compact disc, as well as a book. The recent news of our first great-grandchild's imminent arrival makes this book even more appropriate.

My own family history fades into myths and half-truths after four generations. One great-grandfather, a Petty Officer on H.M.S. Captain, the first British iron-clad warship, perished with most of the crew when she capsized on her maiden voyage in the Bay of Biscay. The crew had looked with apprehension at the revolutionary design of a huge circular gun turret amidships, which shipped water as it rolled. Most of them had prudently made their wills and said their last farewells before embarking.

Another great-grandfather, a mate on a collier taking Newcastle coals to Portsmouth, fell off the gang-plank whilst drunk, and drowned when his sea-boots filled up, but not before siring ten children. His youngest son, my grandfather, became a coal merchant in Portsmouth and never drank alcohol.

These memoirs resulted from a return trip to England after twenty years in Australia. My wife Jill and I decided to see the many places we had lived in, and as both sides of the family were associated with the Royal Navy, we had moved around the country quite frequently, and had sufficient relatives to make an interesting personal Odyssey. We asked an elderly aunt where we had come from, and although she did not know for sure, she mentioned that Grandfather Jelliffe had fossicked for ancestors around the Selsey area in Hampshire near Portsmouth, where he had spent all his life. The local vicar referred us to the church records in Chichester cathedral.

In an oak-panelled room, in the parish records office, we sat on old leather chairs, trying to keep mousy quiet as our excitement mounted, ignoring the frowns of elderly scholars doing genealogical research for paying customers. Previous enterprising investigators had made an index of names from the numerous records returned annually by the parish church wardens over the last four hundred years. We knew that the spellings of that illiterate age were variable, and looked up all combinations and variations of Jelliffe we could think of, including the name Jolliffe which is common on the nearby Isle of Wight.

We found all our names came from four small villages by the mud flats of the huge tidal basin of Chichester harbour: Sidlesham, Apuldram, Chidham and Bosham. We had just visited the latter, as my wife had been there as a child. I had felt strangely at home there and found it was indeed my ancestral village. It is the haunt of the sailing fraternity, and the highest tides come up the main street so that many of the lower lying houses have a high stone across their back doorways to prevent flooding.

It has a church which appears on the Bayeux tapestry depicting King Harold's departure to fall prisoner to William of Normandy, who later defeated him at the battle of Hastings. There, King Canute is said to have unsuccessfully told the tide to turn back, thus demonstrating to his sycophantic subjects that he did not have divine powers. [Cars parked unsuspectingly close to the water's edge today suffer the same fate.] His daughter drowned in the mill stream and was buried in the little church where a stone coffin was excavated last century. On a lighter note, Sir Winston Churchill said of Sir William Bosham, on his entry to Parliament, "What an extraordinary name, neither one thing nor the other!"

The secretary gave us three brown paper parcels, the records from each parish church, tied with red ribbon, and containing a bounty of parchment and faded papers. The earliest decipherable ancestral name was in 1538, thirteen generations ago. We were able to follow the line down to the cut-out date of 1837, when all such records became centralised in Somerset House in London, which we later visited. As we found more and more ancestors, and also some of their wills, our excitement grew. The elderly gentlemen at the other tables "harrumphed" reproachfully, as we waved parchment and paper at each other.

I've found great-great-uncle William. Look what happened to poor little Anne, the latter having been left an orphan at fifteen, and then having two illegitimate babies, both dying in their first week of life. Every year, during the winter storms, there was a burial of an unknown sailor washed ashore. Wives, constantly childbearing, usually did not last long, with a high maternal and infant mortality, but there were records of some tough elderly women who long survived their husbands. We found the names of the wives, and at last knew more of the family genetic pool, but the only details of the mens' occupations were single words, "corn-merchant, yeoman or mariner". We would never know their histories. Having myself lived through extraordinary medical and sociological changes in the last sixty years, I decided to document my own history for the next thirteen generations.

I was born on Easter Sunday, 22 April 1928, at 46 Sneath Avenue, Golders Green, London, to Dorothy Margery née Hebb, and Reginald Eric Victor Jelliffe, naval stores officer at the Admiralty. From three to six years old, I lived in Malta, followed by ten years in Moore Park, fifteen miles north-west of London, attending Northwood Preparatory, then Merchant

Taylors' School. In 1943, my father, in charge of fuelling the fleet to invade Fortress Europe, moved to Portsmouth where I attended the Technical College for two years, I then studied medicine at the Middlesex Hospital Medical School, London, qualifying with Honours in November 1950.

On 2 June 1951, between two six months resident doctor jobs at the Middlesex Hospital and St. Mary's Hospital, Portsmouth, Jillian Fletcher and I were married in Sunningdale church, south of London.

We then spent four years in Nigeria: two eighteen month tours as a medical officer in Azare, Kano and Kaduna, and one year as anatomy lecturer at Ibadan University. Then we returned to England for one year each as Casualty Registrar Nottingham General Hospital and Surgical Registrar at Shotley Bridge Hospital, Consett Co. Durham, before emigrating to Australia in 1959. After two years as medical superintendent of Goondiwindi Hospital, Queensland, we finally moved to Coffs Harbour on the NSW coast as a general practitioner, and, except for five years as hospital superintendent from 1983 to 1988, I remained so, retiring from practice in 2004. I continue my interest in medicine as a part-time lecturer in medicine with the Rural Medical School with up to 30 students; I also examined applicants for visas as required by the Department of Immigration, and occasionally assisted the surgeons in the private hospital.

We have four sons: Michael, ex-missionary pilot in Papua New Guinea, now returned to Australia; Peter, an environmental consultant who died unexpectedly in 2003 aged 49; John who was an air traffic controller and also has a lychee farm north of Brisbane; and Rick who is an expert in computer publishing. Eight grandchildren and one great-grandchild complete the picture.

Here then is a glimpse of my life and the 20th century as I knew it. It has to rely on my fading memory banks, and so is frequently anecdotal, with the minimum of philosophical thought. It has been a fascinating time when medicine has changed from an art mixed with black magic, to a scientific technology. But it is still inexact and contains an air of mystique which the human mind seems to need to protect itself against the cold and often harsh facts of medical science. This, then, is the story of a medical sparrow, flitting into the Great Hall of Life, observing the lives, joys and calamities of his fellows before making his own final exit.

Chapter 1: CHILDHOOD

My mother was one of Grannie Hebb's five children. The first three were large boys, born dead after prolonged labours. The medical practitioner at the turn of the century had little experience of what is now known as interventional obstetrics. He stood at the foot of the bed with his watch chain visible on his waistcoat, and gave verbal but no practical assistance whilst Grannie laboured in vain. Death in labour for mother or child, no matter what the social level, was common. The novels of the era like Oliver Twist highlight this. It was the custom for the widower to look around at the funeral for a successor to bring up his children.

Grannie finally produced my mother, also a large baby, who survived to marry my father and have three live boys herself, before dying of breast cancer aged 38. She had a little sister, Winnie, whose sweet face and cascading blond hair looks out from a few remaining family photographs. She died at sixteen of acute appendicitis.

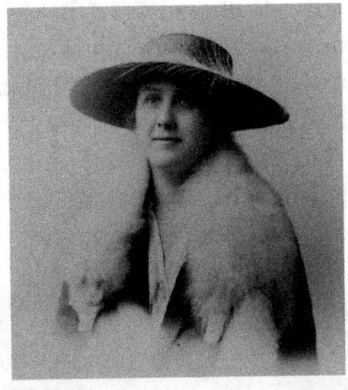

Mother - Dorothy Margery nee Hebb

The country doctor stood at the foot of the bed and said, "If she is no better in the morning, we will have to get her to the hospital." This was at the time of the postponement of King Edward's coronation, following his successful appendectomy, which was then a novel procedure. The morning was too late for poor Winnie.

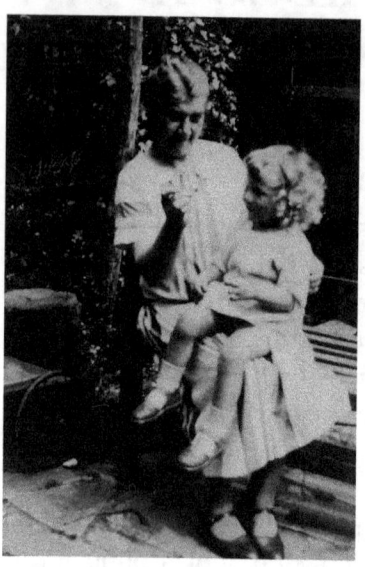

'Grannie' Hebb with a young Robin

I have no personal recollections of my maternal grandfather Major Hebb. His photographs, in the uniform of the Royal Army Service Corps, polished Sam Browne belt and riding boots, holding a little stick under his arm, stare out at us in Singapore, Ashanti and South Africa, reminders of the Victorian expansion of the British Empire. He also bears an uncanny resemblance to my third son John.

My earliest memory is of Malta, where my father was posted when I was three. Black plumes waved over black horses drawing a black carriage past glaringly white houses under a hot Malta sun. The deep, mournful tolling of a church bell mingled with the sorrowful cries of black-clad women. "It's a funeral, dear. Someone has gone to Heaven," said my Maltese nurse, Helen Mizzi. "It's a funny way to go," were my four year old thoughts.

The teddy bear incident also looms large in my memory. We had been on a picnic to Hagiar Qim, on the edge of some cliffs, surrounded by prickly pear cacti, the site of one of the oldest megalithic temples in the world. I left my

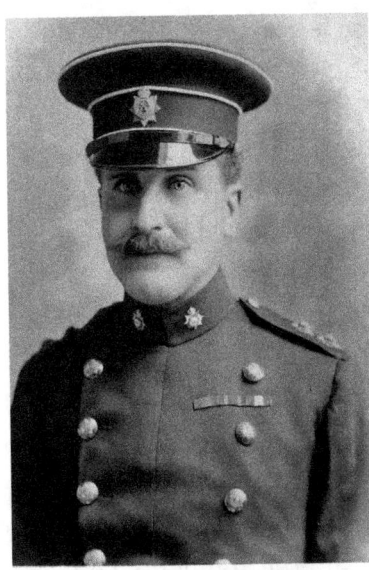

Grandfather - Major James Hebb, MC, RASC 1898

Teddy amongst the enormous monoliths and my father could not find him. He bought another, pulled one glass eye out, my brothers jumped on it, and to give it its full authentic smell, moistened it with a little urine. But they could not fool me. I knew it was not my Teddy, although I learnt to love him almost as much.

There was a beach called Ghain Tuffiya which was ten miles long with a mountain at one end, and fishermen pulling a cartfull of huge fish big enough to make a meal of me. On a later trip, aged twenty-six, I visited the same beach, about a hundred yards long, with a slight rise at one end and fishermen pulling a small cart with fish the size of my arm.

My only other Malta memory was of the P&O liner returning to England. My brothers, five and seven years older than I, had been discussing boomerangs and told me that if I threw my beret over the side, it would return. I still remember the sight of that blue hat passing

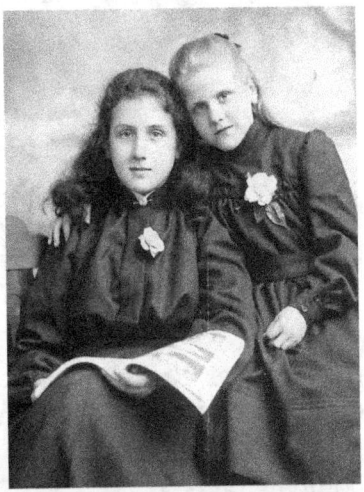

Mother - Dorothy with sister Winnie, about 1910

rapidly astern. That was my first lesson in the ways of the world. The next was when I offered my brother the last chocolate biscuit, and he took it.

We arrived back in England from Malta in 1934 and my mother died soon after. My memories of her are of a large and cuddly smiling figure with a special perfume smell, but I had lost close contact with her during her illness and frequent disappearances to hospital. Grannie Hebb looked after me and spoilt me as the last of her three grandchildren whilst my father spent his days working his way up the civil service ladder as a naval stores officer. He would arrive home about 6 p.m. with stories of the internecine fights between the branches and tell me about the iniquities of "Mr. Griffith at the Offith".

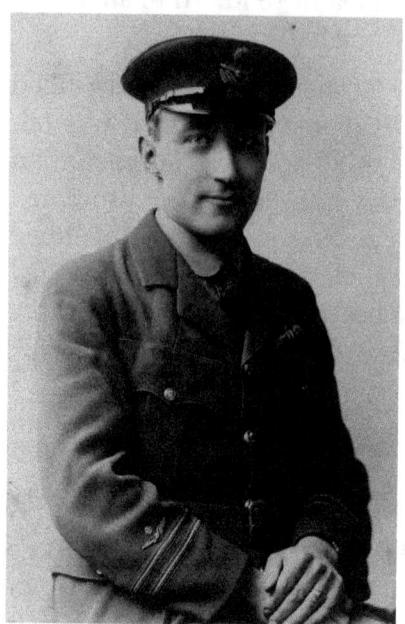

Father - Reginald Eric Victor Jelliffe

He had taken out a mortgage on Meadowbank, a large new house in Moore Park, near Rickmansworth, fifteen miles northwest of London. It was close to Merchant Taylors' school, a guild school started by Edward IV in the fifteenth century. Before the war started, this had been farsightedly relocated from Charterhouse Square in London fifteen miles away to the green belt. The old school was badly damaged in the first bombing raids.

The school motto, Concordia parvae res crescunt, meaning "together little things flourish", greets newcomers on the impressive gates. The playing fields are large, well able to cope with several hundred boys, and the main drive is half a mile long. My two elder brothers were enrolled, and I was booked for a later year, fortunately getting an entrance scholarship, as my father had only a small income. In retrospect, I wonder if those who allocate scholarships realise the profound effect such faith in the recipients has on their lives, and certainly mine. A later scholarship to my medical school enabled me to become a doctor.

We spent most summer holidays with my other grandparents, Thomas and Ellen, living in a tiny terrace house in Southsea, the residential part of Portsmouth. My two cousins, Denis and Raymond, and their parents also crowded into the three bedrooms. My only uncle Harold was in Customs and Excise, and, having learnt to throw his voice as a singer, was a ventriloquist, or so we thought. He told hilarious stories and could make parrot noises come from the trees, and anguished cries for help from inside pianos, whilst reading his paper.

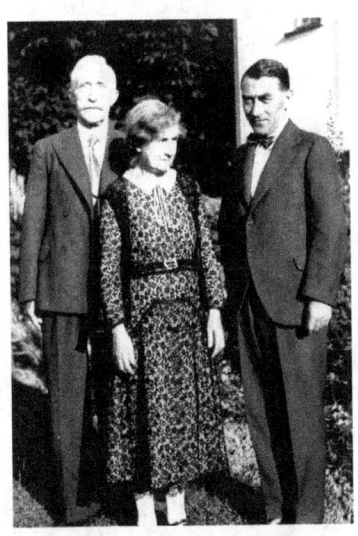

Grandperents- Thomas and Ellen Jelliffe with my father, 1936

Grandfather Jelliffe was a straight-backed, rather stern man, with a large white handlebar moustache, who spent time every morning putting spit and polish on his gleaming black shoes, sharpening a razor-blade on the inside of a glass, catapulting stray cats from the tiny back garden or telling stories of his time in the peace-time Army before becoming a civilian clerk to the Royal Engineers. As a young man, he played the banjo and loved the stage, reciting music-hall monologues flawlessly, tap and clog dancing, and even appearing in an early film. Unlike some of his grandchildren, he had beautiful copperplate writing. He had had an unhappy childhood with a violent drunken mariner father, and ran away from home aged 14 to work in a pawn-shop. Not surprisingly he hated alcohol. He cooked us chips for breakfast and drank his cup of tea in the manner of a filter feeder, sucking the layer of milk off his moustache in noisy appreciation.

Grandma drank tea out of her saucer with her little finger raised in an elegant manner if it was too hot. She was a quiet but tough lady who determinedly pushed her two sons up the socioeconomic ladder with education her top priority. She was very religious, and I suppose this was why my father disliked church.

Sunday evenings tended to be boring, as the only game we could play was "Birds, beasts and fishes", naming as many as possible for each letter of the alphabet. The BBC radio was also dull on Sunday, which was not a day of levity. Today's openness and the types of television program would have devastated her. As a young woman, she would travel by train to and from London on a Friday, to sketch the latest fashions in hats. The Portsmouth milliners would have the new hats ready for sale on Monday.

In a letter to his mother, my father showed his devotion to and appreciation of his mother's efforts. Having just passed an entry examination to the civil service aged 19, he wrote:

"Nevertheless, Mum, however much I have worked, whether little or not, I could not have passed, had not the opportunity been presented

to me. No-one knows how deeply grateful I am to you; I am happy not to pass for myself alone, but that you and I may think that you have not striven in vain. If I do as well by my children (at present a very doubtful proposition) the Jelliffes will be heads of the land. Now I have a ripping position (thanks to you and Pa alone, dear !).

I am wondering, Mum. I have about two pounds and seven shillings by me. Ought I or oughtn't I to buy a new suit (a cheap one) to turn up 'swank' in my new office? You know, the first impression carries a long way. In Clapham, there are some 'remnant' suits, about twenty five shillings. Do advise me, Mum. You know, the doctor swanks his ability to a new district by the parade of a gorgeous carriage and pair."

Or a Mercedes in this day and age.

And in a letter to his brother Harold, he wrote:

"How the blue blazes I managed to excel myself is a matter for conjecture. I do deserve it. I worked hard enough, at least in getting up early. I denied myself the Sports Club and Cricket Captain, to some purpose, I think now. I know you are all happy. Poor old Pa has his happiness now. He can swank to J.Watson, Jonathan Blake and others and say I have at last passed an exam on the list. Have you ever thought what a wonderful manager Mum is? I think I grow prouder and prouder of my dear little mother and dear old Dad!"

My father was the main focus of my childhood life. He would bath me and while putting me to bed, tell me stories of his time in the Royal Naval Air Service in World War I. During his training outside London, he started with free flight balloons.

A long rope trailed from the basket as a height control. If the balloon became too low, more of the rope's weight was taken by the ground and vice versa, keeping the height reasonably constant. This tended to damage the telephone lines of south London, prompting queries as to whose side he was on. There was a girls' school close by the final landing point, and with skill, luck and the right wind, landing could be achieved in the school grounds, ensuring an admiring crowd of pretty girls, help with packing up the deflated balloon and a good tea. The trick was to let the balloon down gently by pulling an emptying valve, which was opened completely when settled safely on the ground. A heavy landing resulted in a half-mile bounce out of the school grounds into less acceptable areas including a sewage farm.

He had been stationed in the north of Scotland, flying airships over the North Sea, protecting the Scottish fishing fleet from U-boats. He saw only one during his service years, raced towards it at his full speed of 50 mph ready to drop his one bomb, but it submerged in time. Perhaps there is a happy family in Hamburg today whose survival is due to his lack of pace. The airships were of the non-rigid type, unlike the German Zeppelins. Three long gas bags were fully inflated to keep their shape intact, and it was with considerable amusement, when learning anatomy later, that I realised that the male organ uses the same pattern.

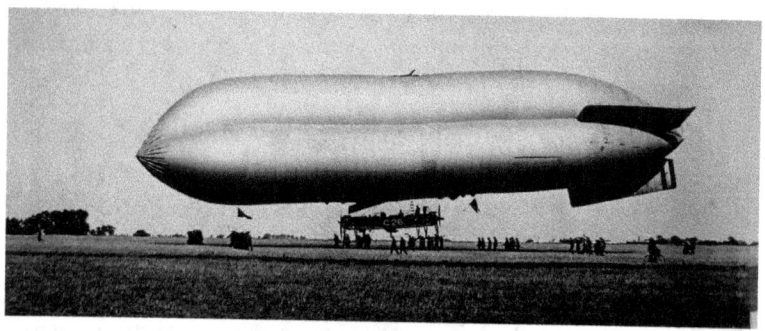

Father's airship, 1917

I will quote verbatim part of an article he wrote, illustrating the adventurous and dangerous nature of his war service and the effect it had on my imagination and a desire to take to the skies.

"It was with dismay that I found myself appointed to airships as a probationary pilot, the existence of which I had overlooked; at that time I could only call to mind the short and ill-fated lives of the Beta and other pre-1914 types, including the Mayfly, which in fact never did.

"Early in 1917, I was posted to Longside, seven miles from Peterhead, to fly coastal airships. These were trefoil in cross section with internal rigging and had a long car suspended underneath, which held in order a 150 hp Sunbeam engine, a large petrol tank, compartments for coxswain, pilot, passenger (or water ballast), W.T. operator, engineer, and finally another large petrol tank for the second engine, which was at the after end. Communication was by walking along the rail outside and ducking under the elevator control wires.

"Before qualifying as pilot of this larger airship, we had to serve a period as coxswain. Flying early one May morning at 1500 feet off Rattray Head, I was much concerned to hear the pilot behind me shout above the noise of the engines, 'We're on fire!' and to see flames streaming from the port side of the for'rd engine. Without rehearsal, we did all the right things, racing up the engine, turning off the petrol tank and squirting Pyrene over the flames, which were extinguished before the wooden engine bearing struts caught alight. What had happened was that vibration in the for'rd engine had fractured the solid pipe from petrol tank to carburettor, and a blow-back through this had set alight the flowing petrol. Flexible petrol leads were used thereafter!

"The Aberdeen fishing fleet had faith in airship protection, of which we were not slow to take advantage. Returning from night flights we became adept at flying slowly, head to wind, over a returning trawler and letting down a canvas bucket, which, having been filled with fish, was hauled up, whereupon we hurried back to a really fresh fish breakfast."

Very recently, I learnt from an elderly German, that U-boats would come alongside these same trawlers and peacefully exchange schnapps for fish.

After the war, he was offered a commission in the newly formed RAF, still flying airships, now of the rigid type, but instead, joined the Admiralty, the civilian branch of the Navy. This was fortunate for both him and my own conception as he lost many friends in the disastrous crash of the airship R101 on its way to India and the far corners of the then British Empire, to show off the latest technology before it had been adequately tested.

In those pre-antibiotic days, I had many attacks of sore throats, becoming delirious with high temperatures when the world changed from smooth surfaces to enormous wrinkles, "crinkly custard" is my wife's description, and my arm would change size from huge to minute in an instant. Childhood is not always the happy state depicted in television butter advertisements where mother and daughter run joyously hand in hand through fields of daisies, their glossy hair bouncing up and down in unison. It was then a time for gaining immunity by contracting childhood illnesses. The only visits to the doctor were for the dreaded tetanus and diphtheria injections and smallpox immunisation by a little scratch on the shoulder, allowing us the privilege at school of wearing a piece of red thread proudly around the tender area, never punched by fellow students.

Unfortunately, I had contracted amoebic dysentery in Malta and had to spend two weeks in the Tropical Diseases Hospital soon after arriving back in England. Here, I was introduced to the antiseptic smell which pervades every hospital, hated by those with unhappy memories, but to me a familiar part of my life. In those pre-antibiotic days, treatment was by a course of retention enemas, which I put up with, enjoying the "brave little boy" image. Successfully cured, the doctor gave my father a diet sheet and told him to keep me on it for three months.

Unfortunately, he misunderstood and I was kept on it for three years. It was a strange diet. Ice cream, sausages and most confectionery were forbidden, but I was to have a banana daily. My two elder brothers became adept at eating their own luxuries out of my sight. Exactly three years later, the diet ceased and I enjoyed ice cream and chocolate again for the next four years before war was declared.

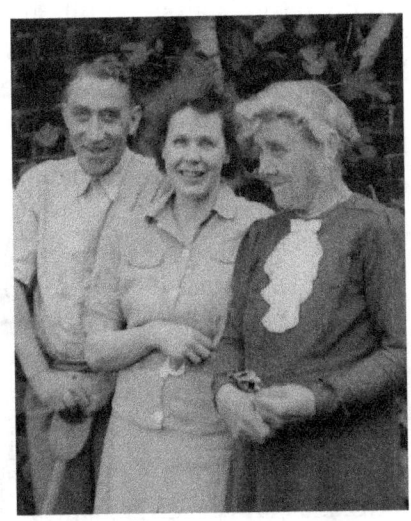

Father Reginald Jelliffe with Step-Mother 'Tim' & Grannie Hebb

The Wall's ice cream man tricycled along our road, with a large insulated box on the front, ringing his bell for customers. A penny bought a delicious Snofruit or Snocream pushed out of a triangular tube and eaten quickly before it melted and dripped stickily on my baggy short trousers. Best value were the tuppenny vanilla slices crunched between wafers. Fourpenny chocolate coated ices were usually too dear for my sixpence a week pocket money, and were the province of visiting uncles or Godfathers, whilst the sixpenny tubs, eaten with a little wooden spoon, were poor value for money in my opinion, but were favoured by the more genteel female callers.

My Godfather, Uncle Eric, was a quiet lugubrious bachelor who always brought me packets of uninteresting barley sugar. Brother Tony's was much more fun, with interesting chocolates and a turn of phrase which had us in fits of juvenile laughter. He was called Uncle Pay, the paymaster in my father's airship unit, and called me "Rob the Dibber" after seeing me dibbing holes in my vegetable garden for lettuces. Wartime later put a stop to chocolate, ice cream and bananas completely.

My father and his friends smoked cigarettes continually, as did my stepmother, whom he married when I was 14. They were mostly Player's Navy with a picture of a rather appropriately named bearded British Jack Tar on the packet, or Wills Woodbines, whose very name symbolised a natural product. My father used names such as "gaspers" or "coffin nails" little realising the consequences of having one in his mouth for most of the day, lighting one from the preceding stub. He died of lung cancer aged 64, a great friend had a stroke at an earlier age and my stepmother wheezed like a litter of kittens. Every room had neatly lidded cigarette boxes and everyone had a flat cigarette case in their coat pocket or handbag, birthday or retirement presents in silver plate engraved with their names. The first action with visitors was to offer a cigarette.

My father once calculated how much he would have saved without nicotine, and at the age of eight, I was a sufficiently mercenary brat, on sixpence a week pocket-money, to decide not to take it up. However, I appreciated the cigarette card in each packet, which I collected and "swopped" to build up the fifty card sets, sticking them into the albums which the tobacco companies conveniently provided for a penny each. Every few months, a new series appeared, Flags of All Nations, Aircraft of the World, Tennis and Film Stars, Types of Dogs. In a way, I must have encouraged the adults to smoke more to try to find the rarer cards, the Hawker

Hart, Bette Davis or the Irish Wolfhound. Years later, an old Gladstone bag was discovered in my nephew's attic which contained several thousand cards and thirty albums with my name on them. I had the incredible experience of reliving childhood memories after sixty-five years.

My first school was Northwood Preparatory School, all male, known affectionately as "Terry's" after its founder. There I stayed till I was twelve, moving steadily up from class to class, an unspectacular student who preferred to stay at home and look after my pet rabbits and make model aeroplanes, than take part in any of the usual sports of cricket and soccer. I enjoyed cricket when it was forced upon me, but I was usually last man to bat, if the captain had not already decided to declare and deny me the opportunity. My father was educating his three sons on a shoe-string and I never had any games equipment until much later, which probably had a dampening effect on any enthusiasm for sports.

My brother Tony had been making scale model aircraft, mostly from Frog and Skybird kits, and I, aged eight, became adept in creeping into his room when he was away, and zooming them about with my hands. Due to damage to an Armstrong Whitworth Scimitar of which he was very proud, the time had come for me to make my own. These I carved out of pieces of balsa wood. When supplies ran out, in the middle of the war, I cycled ten miles to the de Havilland factory at Hatfield, and collected a huge bundle of cast off pieces from the manufacture of the wooden Mosquito aircraft. This was arranged by my father who was then dealing with airframes for the Fleet Air Arm.

Besides building model aircraft, I was an avid photographer, armed with a simple Bakelite Brownie camera using 127 black and white film. Colour photography was in its infancy and the standard 35 mm camera was a German format, yet to sweep the world. I developed my film in a spiral light-proof tank which I loaded in the darkest place in the house, the laundry cupboard where the clothes were kept airing. I made direct prints on silver bromide paper loaded under the negatives in glass-fronted frames in subdued light. No dark room was needed as the emulsion was very insensitive, and the frames had to be exposed to direct sunlight for several minutes. The camera had a fixed focus and a simple shutter mechanism. Like chocolate and bananas, photographic film disappeared when war was declared.

I usually cycled to school five miles through partly wooded countryside alongside the railway line. When the bicycle was in need of repairs, I walked to the station between the leafy corridor of chestnut trees and front hedges or sandstone walls, before running to catch the local train for the four minute trip from Moore Park and Sandy Lodge to Northwood. Thin bars of Nestlé's chocolate with fledglings peeping out of a bird's nest embossed royally on their red packets tempted me from penny slot machines on one platform, whilst near the Northwood station exit, a sweet shop sold sherbet packets to be sucked out with licorice straws. It was then a delightful run to school, on a footpath whose flagstones "plinked" musically under foot.

I started a diary at one stage, but only got as far as "Sick at Hall's party", from overeating, like many other little boys, past, present and future. Cream cakes, sherbet and parties with sufficient food to induce nausea vanished soon after the outbreak of war, and our diet became much healthier, with minimum fats and meat, but always enough bread and vegetables.

On Armistice Day, we marched with other schools to a parade in front of the war memorial to sing moving hymns. *'Oh God, our help in ages past'* meant little to me except the phrase, *'time like an ever rolling stream'* which touched a cord, a brief glimpse of eternity.

The threatening international situation of 1938 was above our heads, but we sensed the anxieties of the teachers, especially a handsome male teacher and his pretty little blonde colleague, to whom he became engaged, much to our delight.

The abdication of King Edward VIII had us all singing a modified Christmas carol in a disrespectful manner:

Hark, the herald angels sing,

Mrs. Simpson's pinched our King.

Mrs. Simpson, awful woman,

Edward's gone and George is coomin.

Naturally, the war brought many changes. We were issued with gas masks, which we were admonished to take everywhere. We had great fun attempting to talk whilst wearing them, and making rude noises with the rubber sides. They were kept in smallish cardboard boxes slung over our shoulders, which quickly became the repository for other boyish necessities, pet mice or half-eaten apples. Eventually there was no room left for the original contents, and like a cuckoo chick evicting its foster-brother, the gas mask was left out. We had identity cards to be carried always, which, like the gas masks, were soon left at home, forgotten except for the identity number. Mine was easy to remember, DENS 131-3, conjuring up unlucky teeth.

We had to maintain blackout conditions at night, with not a crack of light visible, in case it should be seen by marauding German bombers, which might home in on us personally. We made wooden frames to fit the windows exactly, papered them over with several layers of newspaper pasted together, and painted them black. The bicycles had hoods with slits on their headlights, as did the cars, most of which were soon jacked up with their batteries removed for the duration of hostilities.

Air raid wardens came round inspecting for chinks of light, and "Put that light out" became a familiar night cry. Walking at night was hazardous and we were exhorted to eat plenty of carrots for night vision. "Cat's Eyes" Cunningham, an ace night fighter pilot was our example, but it turned out to be a ploy by the Ministry of Agriculture to consume a temporary over-production of carrots.

The local golf club was a huge stately home which had been built at the time of the "Southsea Bubble", a previous century's stockmarket collapse. Alongside some bunkers there were tunnels leading to deep underground storage pits lined with brick, into which we would crawl and drop stones to estimate their depth, and check for enemy agents. The course had concrete blocks placed on the fairways to confound enemy gliders, and a local rule stated that in the event of German paratroopers landing during a game, a marker was allowed to be placed so that the game could be continued when the fighting had ceased. Sheep grazed on these sacred links, making more hazards than normal, and changing many a handicap. Sheep do not understand the word "fore".

At the age of twelve, I enrolled at Merchant Taylors School, and found myself in the science section, learning English, History, Geography, Mathematics, Physics, Chemistry, Biology and one language, French. A typical school day started at 7.30 a.m. with a quick wash and a change of shirt and pants three times a week. Breakfast was a cup of tea, with toast and Marmite spread over a very thin layer of Stork margarine, which got thinner as rationing increased.

I usually walked the mile to Merchant Taylors, a satchel over my shoulder. We gathered in the Great Hall where the headmaster, N. P. Birley, gave us his exhortations and announcements. His educational principle was, 'It does not matter what you teach them, as long as they find it difficult', which was a way of making us learn to think.

We had a short mid-morning break and a communal lunch in the large dining hall. This was a basic but nutritious meal, the contents of which I have completely forgotten, except rice pudding, my favourite. School finished at 4 p.m. and we took our homework back, which took about an hour to do in the evening.

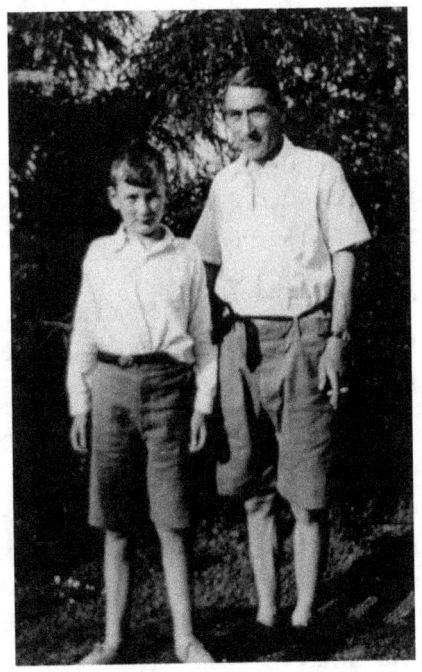

Robin with father, 1940

We had a wide spectrum of teachers. Johnny Fryer, tall and fierce, taught French and German and was held in great respect, awe and sometimes fear. In retrospect he was soft-hearted but had developed an excellent technique for self-preservation atschool. He ruled his class with an iron will, partly on the totally unfounded rumour that he was no longer allowed to use the cane because he had once nearly killed a boy. Certainly, he never did, and it was only used with due ceremony by the headmaster for terrible crimes. We believed that he had been a spy in Germany in the first war, and had received a wound on his bottom, which had a metal plate in it. There was always a hushed silence when he entered and sat down, but we never heard the sound of tin on wood.

Punishment was by "lines", the writing out of a hundred or more of such phrases as "I must not throw paper darts". No pupil was ever slapped or physically attacked. Johnny Fryer could see which pupils were hopeless at French and had a "rubbish heap" at the back, so that the abler boys would not be held back in their work. Academic level playing fields had not yet been invented.

A small overactive Welsh clergyman taught us scripture prancing about the classroom. "Man," he shouted, with a very strong accent, "is not a cosmic microbe." Apart from reading about numerous bloodthirsty Old Testament wars, thinking how tired Moses must have felt to hold up his arms for such long battles, we had very little formal scripture teaching.

As the war progressed, the younger male teachers were conscripted and we had the first woman teacher to enter our masculine territory. She taught us English, and we used to giggle at her, with her hair in a bun, and thick glasses, the classic schoolmarm, at least fifty years old and therefore ancient. She was intensely enthusiastic, trying to teach poetry to a group of adolescents, who were looking enviously out of the window at the sixth form practising at the cricket nets.

We studied Macbeth and Wordsworth that year, and I now realise what an excellent job she did, for I can still quote many of that tragedy's famous speeches and learnt to love the flow of the English language.

The junior school paraded as Boy Scouts for one afternoon each week in a large hall across the quadrangle, where the seniors practiced marching. It was full of the accoutrements of scouting, charts of knots on the walls, stacks of staves and encouragement everywhere to gain further badges, and to Be Prepared. Wearing our Baden-Powell hats, long socks and shorts, scarves tied with toggles, plaited leather rings, and shirts emblazoned with as many badges we could earn without too much effort, we paraded in Patrols. I was in the Peewits and then the Squirrels.

We held our scout staves in the right hand, shaking hands with the left to demonstrate our preparedness with the right. We swore to be "Trusty, loyal and helpful, brotherly, courteous and kind, obedient, smiling and thrifty, and clean in body and mind". We learnt how to make stretchers with our staves, to bivouac, set up tents and tie an assortment of interesting but mostly useless knots. I can still tie a perfect short sheep shank.

Every year, we went on a mid-summer camp. The tents were checked and last year's earwigs shaken out of the musty ground sheets and sleeping bags. We took an assortment of billy cans, frying pans, paraffin lamps, and the all important entrenching tool with which we dug latrines. The camps were held in the rolling green Buckinghamshire countryside, in a cooperative farmer's field which we had promised to return to its pristine state. A small river ran through the bottom of the meadows, and numerous patches of woodland gave us ideal conditions for scout games. Occasionally it rained, when we dripped disconsolately around wood fires which failed to stay alight.

Most memories of scout camp are of bright sunshine, watching the American daylight bombers returning to their bases nearby, often with holes in their wings, or smoking engines, and singing loudly in the long summer evenings around the campfire, although this had to be extinguished at nightfall because of the blackout. The last day, as with most holidays, was an anticlimax, taken up by returning the field and all the equipment to their original state. This meant not only folding damp tents and trying to squeeze their swollen bulk into canvas bags, but also cleaning the pots and pans. Just as we had to light a fire using only two matches, scout lore said the billy cans and frying pans had to have two weeks' greasy soot rubbed off, using only water, paper or leaves and ashes from the fire. Experienced scouts had hidden packets of their mother's household cleaners in their kit bags to ease this final indignity, and could be found with shining utensils and smug, but slightly guilty expressions on their faces.

I enjoyed my time in the Boy Scouts. It encouraged a sense of brotherhood, and knocked out any incipient arrogance. At fourteen, I advanced to the Cadets, known as the Corps, pronounced "Core". We wore World War I uniforms of scratchy khaki material, and the lower quarter of the trousers were bound with puttees, long strips of cloth wound spirally from ankle to mid-calf, to protect the legs from lice in the trenches. Our boots were standard heavy Army pattern and the jackets were fitted with multiple pockets and brass buttons. A peaked cap completed our military appearance. We learnt marching and played with ancient unloaded Lee-Enfield .303 rifles, cleaning them interminably for inspection. We presented and sloped arms, and saluted at every possible occasion.

At the time of the annual Cadets' competition, we were inspected and questioned by an Irish Guards officer, and drilled by a sergeant-major whose peaked cap was tilted so far forward that he had to hold his head at 45 degrees backwards to see properly. I decided to act the exemplary soldier in a dramatic manner. I stamped my feet as hard as possible on stopping and turning, swung my arms stiffly and vigorously, and kept my thumbs exactly in the right position at attention. I answered "Sah" in a stentorian voice, and my salute vibrated at my right eyebrow. I was the perfect ham actor.

I was also very good at aircraft recognition, having carved numerous model aircraft, and made up marks in this new subject. To my surprise, I was awarded my firstever first prize, to the chagrin of another very keen cadet who had worked hard at being the perfect soldier. I felt guilty, but had learnt a valuable lesson. You can succeed with many things if you look as though you mean them.

My elder brother Dick was well into medical school when I entered Merchant Taylors School. I spent many happy hours up the chestnut tree, quizzing him from text books for his anatomy course. "Extensor digitorum longus, origin, insertion, nerve supply, blood supply and action?" He always kept a special eye on his little brother. When we went swimming in the local reservoir, he stayed within rescue distance. I can recall him looking with delight at my eight year old fingers, fascinated by their stubby perfection. Perhaps this was the beginning of his life-long concern for children as patients, for he became a Professor of Pædiatrics and Tropical Medicine.

My other medical student brother, Tony, was very athletic and played rugby football for Merchant Taylors and the medical school teams. He would go out in his football

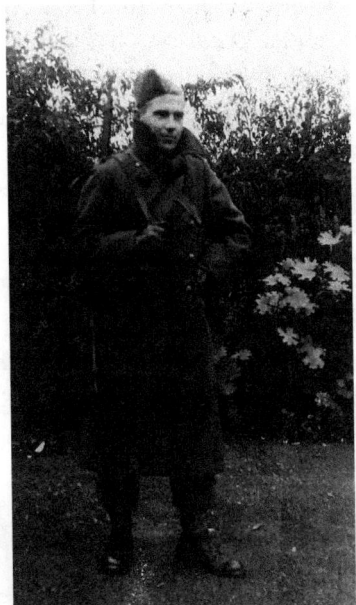

Tony as a Home Guard 1942

shirt and shorts for a five mile run every night, and I would feel privileged to have a cup of steaming Ovaltine, made with wartime powdered milk, ready for his return. He later had a distinguished career in radiotherapy and was a pioneer in chemotherapy at the Middlesex Hospital in London, where we three brothers studied medicine.

Many government departments were moved to safer locations than London when the bombing raids began. My father's branch of the Admiralty, naval stores, went to Harrogate, a rural town of no military or industrial significance, set in the Yorkshire dales. I was left at Meadowbank under the care of Grannie Hebb until my father announced he was remarrying, to his secretary, Miss Simpson, affectionately known as "Tim". She was the antithesis of the wicked stepmother. She took on a ready made family of three boys, at twenty nine, only ten years older than Dick, and was like an elder sister to us all. Besides being an efficient secretary, she was an expert cook whose creations had been photographed for Good Housekeeping magazine. She spoilt us with simple foods elegantly prepared, and seemed to do it all without any effort or leaving a pile of washing up. When I was fourteen, my half-brother Adrian was born, with a very proud brother to look after him. I was no longer the baby, now with responsibilities to bear.

My brother Dick met Pat, a stunning and highly intelligent nurse trainee at the Middlesex Hospital, but the Matron withheld permission to marry until at least one of them had qualified. Despite this injunction, the impecunious pair visited Woolworths for a curtain ring as a temporary wedding ring, and a registry office for a secret marriage. We were all delighted, but Dick and Pat kept the secret from Grannie, as she enjoyed spreading news, which might have got back to Matron. So when they stayed overnight at Meadowbank, they officially used separate bedrooms, on either side of Grannie's room. To complete the charade, Dick tiptoed back early in the morning, whilst Tony flushed both toilets and I ran up and down the stairs, as diversionary noise.

My father used to get very angry, suggesting that Grannie should be told and the apparently shameful arrangement explained. I suspect that Grannie was well aware and, as she and Pat got on extremely well, took no notice. In his early student days, before he did his clinical courses which entailed living in the hospitals, Tony joined the Home Guard. Photographs show him standing jauntily with his rifle slung across his shoulder. He had one moment of glory, when the side of a local country inn was bombed, and the roof collapsed across a bedroom, trapping a couple. He rescued them, but could not be mentioned in dispatches as it was an illicit liaison involving a rather senior army officer. Dick tried to enlist in the Air Force at one stage, but was turned down, as medical students were a reserved occupation, too valuable for canon fodder, as potential doctors.

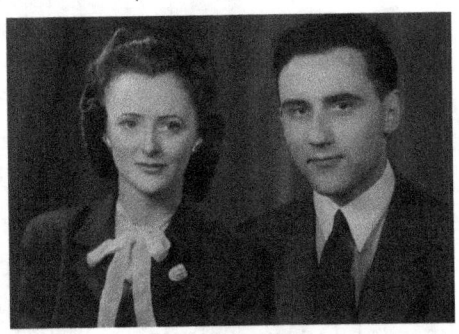

Dick and Pat, 1943

My particular best friend, Edelson, (we traditionally called each other by surnames at school) was in the year below me, but was intelligent enough to be two years ahead. His father was a Russian Jew who had been the equivalent of King's Counsel to the Tsar of Russia, and who had escaped in a sealed train at the time of the Revolution. I soaked up the culture which pervaded their household, in particular the music. At the age of twelve, I had just heard Beethoven's

Fifth Symphony on the radio and was entranced by the slow movement, which I spent days humming, reliving the wonder of that first encounter. My friend's father had all the Beethoven symphonies on 78 rpm records, long before the advent of 331/3 records or CD discs. I remember walking away in a daze from his house, five doors from mine, overwhelmed by the Choral Symphony, even though we had to turn the records over every four minutes. From then on I was hooked on the classics, but I still half expect a pause at the turn-over place in some symphonies.

In 1943, my father was posted to Portsmouth, his home town, in charge of organising the fuelling of the invasion fleet for D-Day. This coincided with my taking the school certificate examination, when I was unlucky enough to catch a viral chest infection. I was given the early sulphonamide drug which prevented pneumonia, but I missed taking the French examination, which was my best subject. The house was sold, and I was enrolled at Portsmouth Technical College to complete my school certificate, and to start my premedical studies in chemistry, physics and biology.

In 1943, my father rented a house easily enough as there had been few holiday visitors to an area which had been badly bombed and was still a priority target. For security reasons, the whole of southern England was sealed off to all except residents, and we needed permits to enter. The house was in Southsea, close to the canoe lake where we had hired paddle boats in happier days. It must have looked like a dock from the air, as a 500 pound bomb landed in it one night, breaking many windows in the adjacent hotels, then occupied by Wrens, the womens' branch of the Navy. My father's office overlooked HMS Victory, Nelson's flagship, which had received a bomb into its dry dock, but the mighty oak timber stood up to the blast better than a modern ship and was completely reparable later on.

I would cycle down the back streets to the college, which was opposite the bombed out shell of the town hall. The whole area was crammed with naval personnel, preparing the fleet for the invasion of Europe. On moonlit nights, ideal for raiding aircraft, my father would take me up to Portsdown Hill overlooking the city. Before the war, a huge cathedral-like cavity had been excavated deep inside the chalk hillside, and vast fuel tanks sufficient to supply the whole fleet five times had been installed. Safe under two hundred feet of solid chalk, pumping machinery delivered it by pipeline to Gosport, opposite Portsmouth. We entered through a small steel gate, and walked a hundred yards underground to sleep on camp beds, in our own private bomb-proof shelter.

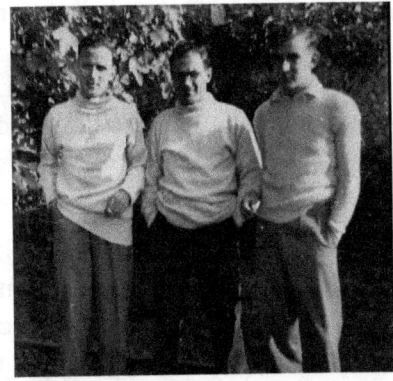

Three brothers - Dick, Tony, Robin

A short cycling distance from Southsea lies Hayling Island, reached by a five minute ferry ride. This is the entrance to Chichester harbour, where I later found my ancestral villages of Apuldram, Bosham and Chidham are situated. Huge rectangular concrete structures, the size of office blocks were being built on the sand flats, to be towed over later to the Normandy beaches and sunk to provide instant harbours. Out in the countryside, every hedgerow had its pile of ammunition, or a bivouac of tanks and army trucks, complete with crews from many nations. Nearer the naval base itself, overlooking the Solent, batteries of anti-aircraft rockets stood ready to annihilate any enemy aircraft, with a barrage which could make a cubic mile of sky lethal with steel fragments. The number of ships in the Solent grew daily.

On D-Day itself, after a night of much air activity, all of them sounding friendly, not the partially unsynchronised hum-hum- hum of enemy motors, I awoke to find the Solent completely empty. Overhead, squadron after squadron of fighters escorting twin engined bombers, and larger aircraft towing gliders headed south for Normandy. There followed a strange quietness, as if the whole coast was holding its breath with only the skylarks and the sea birds audible. Then came the sound of returning aircraft, some limping home with smoking engines and perforated wings and tailplanes. I listened all day to the radio and spent a restless night imagining the desperate conflicts going on a hundred miles away.

Shortly after the invasion, I heard a strange deep-throated pulsating roar and looked out to see a tiny aircraft pass overhead very fast. A few seconds later, the noise stopped followed by a loud explosion. It was the first flying bomb to be fired at Portsmouth. My friend, Scottie, lived at Lee-on-Solent, a village half way between Portsmouth and Southampton, which were both on the track of these weapons. Several times in the middle of a telephone conversation, a flying bomb would roar over and I would then hear it over Scottie's phone line, both waiting for its engine to cut, which would be followed a few seconds later by a thousand kilograms of high explosive hitting the ground. When the firing sites in Brittany were over-run by the Allied armies, no more were launched in our direction and London remained the main target.

With the completion of the invasion of Europe, my father was transferred to Ceylon, now Sri Lanka, to help organise the invasion of Japan, leaving me to lodge at Scottie's mother's boarding house in Lee-on-Solent. It was a pleasant half hour's bicycle ride to catch the ferry across the harbour from Gosport past the rows of ammunition dumps awaiting transit. I studied at Portsmouth College next to the shell of the town hall, which had not survived the air raids. It ran courses in all the science and arts subjects and had girl students, quite a culture shock after my years in boys' schools.

I had had excellent basic training in chemistry at Merchant Taylors school, and had spent hours lying face down on my bed at home, eagerly perusing my elder brothers' textbooks. Apart from lectures, we spent hours in the laboratory, doing more and more complicated experiments with test tubes and Bunsen burners, in particular running through a sequence of tests to identify mystery compounds, which exercise was to occur in our final examination. Like all chemistry students, we made homemade explosive devices, and on one occasion, fired a small metal thermometer case like a rocket out of the window, in retrospect a foolish thing to do in wartime.

Physics consisted of numerous boring lectures, progressing from energy, through optics and magnetism to electricity. Solid state electronics were unknown, and we carried out experiments with grimy pieces of equipment of wood and wire. Small electrical currents were measured by giant dials, or mirrors attached to small magnets reflecting a light beam which would indicate tiny changes in magnetic fields.

Biology was a different story. It was taught by a very elderly lady who was mostly interested in botany for the non-medical students. This formed a very small part of the premedical curriculum. We cut and stained pieces of leaves and plant stems for microscopy, and searched drops of water for organisms with strange names, Pandorina, Euderina and Volvox, scurrying about on the glass slides.

For zoology, we gradually dissected our way up the evolutionary scale, earthworm, cockroach, dogfish, frog and rabbit. The gentle pace of these dissections allowed much socialising, especially with the newly discovered species, girls, who seemed eager to listen respectfully to my sixteen year old dissertations on vertebrate anatomy. I passed chemistry and physics, but was "referred" in biology, which I passed soon after.

I left Portsmouth to begin five years of intensive study at London's Middlesex Hospital Medical School, and moved to lodgings in London. It was time to become a real medical student.

Chapter 2: MEDICAL STUDENT

In a long off-white coat of varying shades of grey, I walked nervously into the anatomy dissecting room with fifteen other new students. These were the first dead persons I had seen, apart from a surreptitious glimpse of Grandfather Jelliffe lying in state under a white sheet three years previously in Portsmouth. The rows of concrete slabs were covered with grey sheets, stained with grease and formalin. Under some were the obvious shapes of full length bodies. Others, less obviously, were arms, legs, trunks and heads. Professor John Kirk, a rawboned Scotsman with a background of missionary work in China, requested our attention.

"You, gentlemen, are at the beginning of your careers. The specimens you are to dissect are at the end of theirs. They have elected, in life, to donate their bodies, after death, to train you to become doctors. The law requires that after one year, they be given a decent burial. Meanwhile, respect them and learn from them."

I joined Martin, Keith and Willie around a sheet, which was whisked away to reveal a large pale female cadaver. The Prosector came over with an encouraging look. He was a recently qualified doctor, studying anatomy in greater detail for the feared "Primary", the basic first part of the post-graduate surgical degree, a reef upon which many a would-be surgical career had foundered.

"You've got breast and axilla" he said and walked to the next slab. "You've got lower limb" and proceeded down the row. "Upper limb", "thorax", and "Hello, Charles, head and neck for your last term."

Martin and I exchanged glances, feigning nonchalance. We unrolled our bundle of instruments and selected a scalpel. The real thing seemed different from the pickled dogfish, frog and rabbit of earlier days.

"Make an incision from here to here," advised our twenty-five year old Father Figure. The scalpel blade slid easily through the crisp skin, revealing a layer of semi-liquid fat. The smell of formalin increased. Blotting out thoughts of this specimen's previous animation, and sobering thoughts of our own ultimate mortality, we continued the dissection down to the axilla.

"You will find the long nerve of Bell beneath that layer of fat, there it is, big as a house, gentlemen," the professor encouraged us in his rolling Scottish accent, a true descendant of the ancestral line of great Edinburgh anatomists.

"And who was Bell?" he asked. Silence followed. The only name I knew to date was Cuvier, a French embryologist not remotely connected with a nerve in the thorax. Time and again in my student career, I was to hear that question, "And who was…?" Later, we students would play a game of one-upmanship in learning more and more abstruse names and syndromes to trump our partners' medical trivia. But Sir Charles Bell was no trivium.

"Over here, gentlemen." From the wall projected a fan of Bell's beautifully detailed original drawings, one hundred and fifty years old. One showed the arm lifted to expose a network of muscles, blood vessels and the legendary long thoracic nerve. Later, this nerve would serve as a landmark in mastectomies, a boundary for removal of cancerous tissues. Damage to it would paralyse an important shoulder muscle and cause a "winged scapula".

"This makes it crystal clear, gentlemen. Sir Charles Bell, a great anatomist."

As the months progressed, the faces of our fellow students became familiar and their characters and abilities emerged. Our brightest was a quietly spoken son of a Welsh miner, on a scholarship; equally intelligent, or perhaps more mature was an exsoldier, a veteran of the Eighth Army in North Africa, married with a young family, on a demobilisation educational grant. The rest of us were of varying degrees of intelligence and ineptitude, hopeless cases having been eliminated by the filter of the First MB examinations in physics, chemistry and biology. There was no quota of the highest 1% of the Higher School Certificate as happens now. We had a wide spectrum of personalities from the quietly religious to the sexually athletic. To a very innocent eighteen-year old, the success stories of the latter group appeared like Arabian Night tales, or the exploits of Don Juan. In retrospect, I fancy that their boasting probably exceeded their prowess, but the fact that such things as they described could and did occur in real life made the hours of patient dissection more entertaining.

After one particularly dishonourable episode, the culprit was called to the professorial study. But Professor Kirk had confused the religious with the randy. "You had better go and talk to your Father," he advised, and was nonplused by the reply, "Righto, I'll phone him straight away."

We progressed down the arm to the hand and fingers, and began to appreciate the respect of our professor for the precision and intricacy of nerve fibres and fine muscles in the appendage that helped raise us above other species. Post-graduate students who appeared from time to time to revise, emphasised the importance of knowing the hand. The livelihood of so many workers with injured or infected hands depended on this knowledge. Without fully functioning hands, they would be relegated to the industrial scrapheap.

We spent two months each on the upper limb, lower limb, thorax, abdomen, brain and head-and-neck. The latter was the most difficult part as we had to dissect inwards, which was easy with a thin object like a limb, but more complicated with the multiple layers of the neck. The students today can use computerised models to build up from the bony structures outwards.

Cramming an extraordinary amount of solid facts was facilitated by the use of mnemonics, short and usually obscene phrases or limericks to aid memory. "Lovely French Tarts Strip Naked In Amiens" represented the structures passing through a long forgotten crevice in the skull, of no real use in later medical practice.

The perennial poem on the nerve to the tongue is enshrinedin the memory of every medical student:-

> *The lingual nerve, it takes a swerve,*
>
> *across the hyoglossus.*
>
> *Said Wharton's duct, "Well I'll be ****ed,"*
>
> *The bugger's double-crossed us!*

"You know more about your Fat Ladies than your anatomy," said Professor Kirk.

The rarest item for dissection was the brain, which rapidly disintegrates after death, and has to be preserved as soon as possible. Much of our studies were from pots, slices and pre-dissected lumps of greyish matter wrapped in cloths soaked in formalin. Some had been prepared with their arteries injected with different coloured dyes, illustrating the areas supplied, useful knowledge in assessing strokes and brain tumours.

Each student possessed a half-skeleton, purchased from the previous class. These genuine bones may have come from India or China and they became our familiar friends. We chalked in red the origins of muscles and the insertions, or lower ends, in blue. Traditionally, green marked the nerves where they touched the bones. We kept the eight wrist bones in our pockets and could identify them by feel alone. Occasionally, whilst studying in the train on the way to work, an obviously human bone would escape but we were never arrested. If our greasy anatomy manual slipped onto the railway carriage floor, it often seemed to open at the picture of the female genitalia, to everyone's embarrassment.

The base of the skull was a favourite area for one-upmanship, full of minute holes through which passed obscure nerves . The Palato-vaginal canal seemed a most unlikely name for one of them. The top of the skull had been sawn off like a hardboiled egg, revealing the asymmetrical grooves made by the great venous sinuses. The asymmetry was supposed, incorrectly, to indicate right or left-handedness, and Professor Kirk had a story to match.

Whilst exploring a cave in Palestine he came across a skull. His archaeologist companion, determined to impress, said it must have been that of a Roman soldier."Yes," said the professor, twinkling his eye, "and a left-handed Roman soldier."

Half way through the course, I decided to visit the operating theatres to see the difference between the live and the dead. Feeling brave, as after all I was a medical student, I entered the quietest theatre, where a nose operation was in progress. A large pair of forceps was thrust up a nose, a disgusting snuffling noise occurred and I slipped to the floor feeling strangely dizzy. This was my first and only theatre faint.

Anatomy showed us the nuts and bolts of the body, whilst physiology gave us an insight into its function. We were fortunate to have Professor Samson Wright, one of the greats of the academic world and author of a standard text-book. He was a short Jewish man, with a chain-smoking habit which ultimately caused his death from heart disease. He came to lectures twenty minutes late, talked politics for twenty minutes and spent the final twenty minutes giving us a lucid dissertation which we remembered for ever.

The politics of the day concerned the controversial attempts by Britain to keep the Jewish refugees out of Palestine. Militant terrorists, or freedom fighters, depending on one's ethnic background, blew up the King David Hotel, shot and were shot at and sometimes hanged. One day, "Sammy" came in and announced that there would be no lecture as "we" had just put one of his friends in jail despite the fact that "we" were generally sympathetic to their cause. Lectures were soon resumed with no ill feelings on either side. Professor Kirk's favourite expression was "crystal clear, gentlemen". Sammy's short lectures were exactly that.

We learnt to "pith" frogs by putting a needle into their spinal cords like miniature matadors to obtain nerve-muscle specimens. The muscles were attached to crude levers and we touched these to smoked paper wrapped around a rotating drum. Electrical impulses stimulated the motor nerves and satisfying patterns appeared on the black paper, to be varnished as a permanent record of that particular amphibian. The rate of stimulation was varied by a simple mechanism, similar to a child's irritating habit of holding a knife blade on a table whilst allowing the other end to vibrate up and down. Later, we ourselves became the guinea-pigs, and inserted fine recording needles into our own muscles, vying with each other to produce one solitary electrical spike, a sign of exquisite muscle control.

The action of nicotine was demonstrated one long afternoon. We were divided into three groups, smokers, occasional smokers and non-smokers, such as myself. The experiment was to demonstrate the action of nicotine in stimulating the production of the anti-diuretic hormone which stops the production of urine. We drank glass after glass of water until we felt bloated and had a maximum urine output. Then we smoked two cigarettes, inhaling to get the full nicotine effect. We non-smokers retched over the basins, the occasional smokers looked green and the smokers watched with ill-concealed amusement. Urine production ceased in the non-smokers for two hours and our first drops were injected into rats, causing them to stop urine production, thus showing the hormone had been produced in sufficient quantities to appear in the urine. We then dispersed homewards, myself on the Underground train without realising the consequences.

As the effects of the nicotine wore off, the kidneys let go the huge overload of water. There are no toilets on the Underground trains, and those at stations are at the end of long, long tunnels. Never, ever, has a comfort station been so well named as I broke my journey in desperation.

Two weeks before Christmas, the pharmacology professor approached our group with a proposition. Would we like to earn £5 by being guinea pigs for a week to test a new type of analgesic? As my total allowance for the month was £8 for food, lodging and transport, this was indeed a princely sum, especially before Christmas. Ten of us were ensconced in a room in the main hospital with beds, armchairs, coffee-making facilities and card-tables, all a student needed for a comfortable few hours. The pain threshold testing apparatus was basic, but ingenious. It was a box, with a hole equipped with a shutter on one side wall. Inside, a light bulb shone its rays through the aperture, the voltage being controlled by a calibrated variable resistance. We blackened our foreheads with burnt cork for constant reliable absorption, placed them against the hole and the lamp was turned on. At first there was just a warm sensation, but when the power was increased to a certain level by the variable control, a twinge of pain was felt. This was the pain threshold. The staff then gave us each an unknown injection and we had our threshold measured at half hourly intervals. Some of us passed out, some looked very happy, and some vomited. We earned our £5.

Later, the professor explained the experiment to us. It was 1948 and the pharmacology industry in Germany was being investigated for useful new drugs. As morphine was in short supply with little access to the opium poppy, the German chemists had been producing substitutes, including the one with which we had been tested, later to become known as methadone.

I have a quirky sense of pride that I was probably the first person in the English-speaking world to try a methadone fix, not that I enjoyed it. I had to return home in a suburban train to Cheam in the middle of winter, with the world rotating around me, and a desperate desire to open the train window for fresh air, vigorously opposed by the other evening travellers. Nowadays, they would have thought me another "junky". The other injections given for comparison were morphine (I vomited), pethidine (I was very happy) and plain water (I was slightly happy, a placebo effect). One student became so pain-free from his dose, that he had blisters on his forehead for the next week. Recently, I told this story to a professor of Pharmacology, who asked after our Ethics Committee's feelings, but of course, such committees were then unknown. No-one had any after-effects nor became addicted, and there was enough money in our pockets to buy better than the usual token Christmas presents.

We also began to study pathology, the abnormal changes in the previously normal. We spent much time in the pathology museum, a large room with an upper gallery, and hundreds of glass and perspex containers on layers of shelves. Inside were the pickled remains of interesting and instructive patients. Hearts, lungs and livers showed us the dangers of smoking, overeating, alcohol and syphilis, remembered as "smoking, stoking, soaking and poking". We suspected that the old pathologists must have been underfed, as most of their descriptions of diseased organs compared them to common edible items, such as sago spleen, bread and butter pericardium, anchovy sauce pus and red current jelly stools. I used to roll around my tongue the splendid description of tuberculous glands, whose contents changed from a pultaceous mass to a grumous fluid.

Some of the exhibits were over a hundred years old, dating back to the early days when the hospital had been started to investigate any and every way of treating cancer. Some of those methods were barbaric such as pouring acid into incisions in a breast cancer, a desperate measure in the days before anaesthetics, surgery, radiotherapy and chemotherapy. A section was reserved for the bizarre, including half the throat of a man who used to earn money in public houses by catching a billiard ball in his teeth, until one day he missed and plugged his airway.

Working in pairs, we got to know each pot and its description intimately, questioning and being questioned. The patients from whom the specimens came, were better known in death than in life. As night fell, the number of pathology students sitting in the museum decreased. Study becomes difficult when surrounded by a thousand ghosts, in a dimly lit room in an eerie silence, however much one disbelieves in the supernatural.

We learnt living pathology in the biochemistry and microbiology departments, peering down microscopes at sections of tissues embedded in little paraffin blocks, sliced thinly and stained with different coloured dyes. I also earned pin money by going around the wards doing blood counts on cancer patients having radiotherapy, or primitive chemotherapy such as nitrogen mustard. The pathologists had no sophisticated automated machines to give multiple results within minutes as happens now, and all tests involved hours at a microscope, counting cells in little squares on the slides.

We also had a lighthearted look at pharmacy, learning the antiquated apothecarie's measurements, minims, drachms and pennyweights, soon to be replaced by the metric system. We ground up chemicals and herbs with pestles and mortars, and learnt to write out long prescriptions. These started with the main constituent, then the secondary substance, then the counter balance and its backup, and finally the flavour and the excipient or pharmacologically inert base. We wrote shorthand Latin phrases, Fiat mist. and Sig: ter in die many of which are still standard, B.D., T.D.S., P.R.N. in time honoured style. Many of the mixtures and ointments carried the names of their function or inventor. Mist. Euthanasia or Brompton's mixture, named after the London Chest Hospital, contained gin, honey, cannabis, and heroin and was used for the terminally ill. Mist. Diabolicus was a disgusting concoction of evil tasting asafoetida and valerian with an agent to cause belching and therefore further prolong the bad taste. It was used for neurotic patients to try to discourage them, but most of them came back for more, on the principle that the worse the taste, the more effective the medicine. The number of truly pharmacologically active substances, either of mineral or botanical origin, could be counted on the fingers of both hands. There was still a lot of black magic and placebo therapy in the late 1940s, now replaced by an avalanche of highly potent medications with equally potent side effects. The thin handbook of pharmacy has been replaced by the therapeutic index tome.

The one hundred and fiftieth anniversary of the founding of the hospital was celebrated by exhibitions in all departments. The physics unit set up a radar microwave beam across a room, focusing it with a garbage can lid onto a coil of steel wool which sparked and crackled. The dangers of cooking a spectator were not fully realised. The one and only electrocardiogram, which lived in the basement, had its three leads attached to a student to demonstrate this new technological wonder. The physiologists attached fine needle electrodes to other students and showed the blips of electrical activity on a cathode ray tube. But neither the anatomy room nor pathology museum were open to the public.

Anatomy, physiology and pathology were the basic building blocks for our medical careers, and took up most of our time, learning fact after fact with no real reference to their future use in medicine. It was only later that the value of going back to basics stood in good stead with difficult clinical cases. I have no recollection of taking the 2nd M.B. examinations except the immediate after-examination feeling experienced by every student, medical or otherwise, of having done badly . I was relieved to find I had, with most others, passed, having underestimated my academic ability and the generosity of the examiners.

Chapter 3: CLINICAL STUDENT

My introduction to the living patient was in the casualty department of the Middlesex Hospital where I spent the first six months of my clinical training. In 1946, many doctors had not yet been demobilised and those that were, were sufficiently senior to be above the humble casualty officers' work. So the students were welcomed as good work horses, and after a short series of demonstrations by the junior doctor, and more importantly, the sister in charge, we were allowed to do more and more complicated procedures.

We were paired off and told to give each other injections after practising on pieces of fruit. Martin, later my best man, hovered nervously at my upper arm, the needle point shaking back and forth touching the skin. Finally, he drove it in, to my surprise at its painlessness and our mutual relief that he had not broken it off in my arm. We were then allowed to attack the patients themselves, both the scared and the stoic, whose welcome philosophy was, "Well, Doc, you've got to learn."

This was in the early days of penicillin, a clear painful solution, golden with impurities, given into the upper buttock every four hours. The first long acting refined penicillin was white and mixed with beeswax. This was solid at room temperature and its bottle had to be placed on the hot steriliser lid to allow it to melt. We would draw it up as quickly as possible into a hot glass syringe armed with a thick needle and rush over to the patient, lying skirt up or trousers down, to inject the treacly fluid before it had a chance to solidify. Sterile abscesses were common as the tissues reacted against the insoluble wax and sometimes required incising later. The advent of long acting procaine penicillin superseded this unpleasant procedure.

We learnt how to give short anaesthetics with nitrous oxide, using five breaths of gas followed by one breath of air. The resulting unconscious state due mostly to the sudden lack of oxygen, was gauged by the degree of blueness of the eyes and nails, really a very hazardous method. It was sufficient for quick incisions of abscesses, or the reduction of dislocated fingers or shoulders. We became adept at local anaesthetics, using injections of Novocaine for the large number of finger injuries which attend every casualty department, lacerations and crushes, and exploring for foreign bodies, from needles to grease from high pressure lubricators.

Sister taught us the arts of stitching and dressing wounds, bandaging, slings and plastering. At night, when the pharmacists had gone home, we dispensed medicines to emergency cases, and met our first amphetamine addicts. We finished our six months term overconfident, thinking we knew everything.

The ensuing year of work alternating in the surgical and medical wards brought us back to earth. It was here that we met the sickest patients with the deadliest diseases. The ordinary hospitals cared for the ordinary cases. The Middlesex Hospital, being a teaching hospital, admitted the most difficult cases, which often meant the most hopeless.

It gave a false idea of medicine and my first encounters with death.

My mother had died of breast cancer when I was six. I cannot remember much about her other than her lying in her bed, deep in a nest of quilted eiderdown. She was often absent having treatment in the Middlesex Hospital. The doctor in Malta, where she first noticed the breast lump, had told her to watch it, a criminal procrastination. It was soon too late for curative surgery and she had radiotherapy as a palliative form of treatment. After she died, I felt vaguely ill at ease, but as Grannie Hebb had looked after me for those last two years, I had bonded well to her. She was always around to comfort and spoil me as the last of her three grandchildren.

There was a short impersonal contact with death at preparatory school. A wild, and in retrospect, intellectually impaired boy in my class was killed whilst playing on a railway line. The headmaster said a few words and we stood in respectful silence for two minutes. The general feeling was a few moments of disbelief, followed by "There but for the grace of God, go I". We had all played near the line and we shrugged it off with a guilty sense of relief that it was not us but he, always a distracting influence, who had gone. He was psychologically disposable. We gave no thought to his grieving parents.

Both my paternal grandparents died in their late seventies and, to a nineteen year old, this seemed an acceptable age to die, "a good innings", we all felt. It was with Leonora that Death hit home. She was one of my first patients, allocated to us as students in the medical ward. We practised taking histories and blood samples, doing clinical examinations and when sufficiently experienced, setting up intravenous drips. We were in the happy-go-lucky stage of studenthood, with examinations just passed and two years to go before the next. We worked with pretty young nurses and urine testing meant retiring to the sluice room to boil up the test tubes with Fehling's solution. "Why don't you slip into something comfortable, like the sluice room?" was a favourite invitation for a dalliance.

Leonora was twenty one, the star pupil of the Royal Academy of Dramatic Art with a personality to match. She had an enchanting smile, limpid brown eyes, a quirky, devastating Jewish sense of humour and disseminated lupus erythematosis. This auto-immune disease was attacking her heart and kidneys and she became breathless when she laughed which was frequently.

She teased me as "her" student and enjoyed the attention she attracted from our all male group. She loved playing tricks, and waited one afternoon until it was time for me to go home, then sprayed me with a bottle of perfume. Naturally, I had to stay until the scent had dissipated, as the train trip home would have caused considerable adverse comments. I found her in tears one morning, and attempted to cheer her up, until she told me her father had just died. I had no idea how to handle the situation and after a quick "sorry", left her to her sorrow as she requested. We were never taught bedside manners, sympathy or how to break bad news, each one an art in itself, the real art of medicine. Hippocrates said, *"Life is short, the art is long, opportunity fleeting and experience fallacious"*.

Even after years of practice, many doctors cannot bring themselves to tell patients the truth about their mortal illnesses. It is the hardest professional duty. Medicine itself is the easier part.

A few months later, I telephoned her sister to ask after Leonora's health, to be told that she had just died. For the first time in my life, I felt a momentary dizzy, sinking feeling, and uncontrollable tears welled up. So much for my tough masculine exterior, I thought. Leonora's death struck home as nothing had before. What a waste! Where was she now? Such a personality could not be gone, but it was.

In our present era, she would have been treated with cortisone and could be alive today. In 1948, there was no such substance. Two biochemicals called Kendall's compound E and F had just been described, later to be called cortisone and hydrocortisone. A minute quantity could be extracted from thousands of animal suprarenal glands. "Analyse, then synthesise " was the basis for pharmacology research. All possible sources for the basic steroid chemical were sought, even the collection of gallstones. Finally, a cheap and inexhaustible supply was found in a type of Mexican yam, and cortisone is now prepared in huge quantities, but too late for Leonora.

Duodenal and gastric ulcers were treated by bland diets. Milk drips through a small nasal tube into the stomach attempted to neutralise excess acid twenty four hours a day . The only medications were atropine-like substances and the antacid mixtures, including a bismuth compound straight from the apothecaries of old. Years later, when the bacterium responsible for peptic ulcer was identified, it was indeed found to be sensitive to bismuth which has made a come back. Many ulcers became resistant to medical treatment and needed surgery, either as an emergency when they ruptured or bled, or the pain became unbearable, or if the outlet from the stomach narrowed with scar tissue. Surgery is rare now, as a result of acid suppressing drugs, and the recognition of the causative bacteria. Most acute ulcers now occur as a result of taking anti-inflammatory drugs for arthritis, and we had only aspirin then.

We were seeing the end of medicine as an art, when physicians treated diseases named after the first doctors to describe them, Addison's, Graves', Parkinson's, Charcot-Marie-Tooth. The prognoses they gave were accurate as they had followed many cases downhill to the post-mortem room, where the clinical signs they had listened to or palpated, were frequently, but not always confirmed. In many cases, there was no treatment of value and we quoted Hilaire Belloc to each other, "... Saying, as they took their fees, There is no cure for this disease."

We accompanied these elderly physicians reverently on the grand rounds. The ward sister ensured that each bed was occupied by a clean patient, tucked rigidly under clean sheets, with all notes up-to-date: pulse, temperature, blood pressure, respirations, bowel action and urine tests. In clean long white coats the registrars had all test results and medication sheets available, and the young resident doctor, or Houseman, carried a tray with knee-jerk hammer, ophthalmoscope, tuning fork (to check for vibration sense) and other simple devices. We students in short white coats stood nervously on the periphery. Each one had his history and clinical examination ready for the moment when the great man in his frock coat would turn to him and ask for his opinion in a gentlemanly manner. He would then expound on the case, the physical signs he heard through his stethoscope, the treatment and, of course, the prognosis, ignoring the patient who was just the Third Person Invisible. This was couched in euphemistic terms which the patient was supposed not to understand, but to which we nodded our heads wisely. Most students hoped to have at least one resident post at their teaching hospital to further their careers, so it was as well to be on the consultant doctor's side. We were also quietly observing their distinctive characteristics for use in the students' Christmas concert sketches.

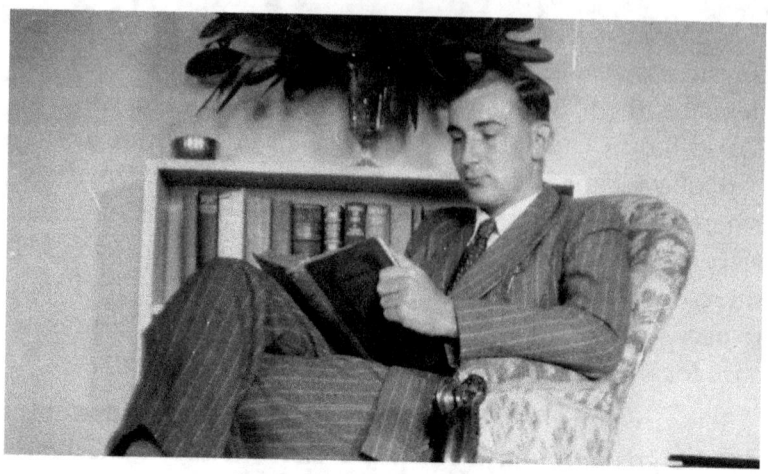

Medical student Robin, aged 21

The surgical wards were completely different. Surgeons were supposed to cure with the healing knife. They frequently turned up in long white coats or sports jackets, and never in frock coats. They tried to live up to the image of "steely eyes and strong steady hands", and succeeded. We had some of the great names in surgical advances on the wards, including the pioneers in breast cancer surgery. Some of the wards were extremely smelly, especially those with prostate cases. Before the days of internal removal by cystoscope, a metal box, which always leaked, was placed on the abdominal wound to collect spillage of urine.

Antibiotics were in their infancy and the odour of infected urine identified the urologist's ward from a considerable distance. Some sisters were adept at sniffing out the pungent smell of early gangrene in infected wounds, as accurately as Customs sniffer dogs searching for heroin at airports. The cleaners saved all the old tea leaves from the huge ward teapots and spread them on the polished wooden floor around the beds, effectively sweeping up dust, unpleasant fluids and hopefully bacteria, whilst acting as an early form of deodorant.

Surgical ward rounds tended to be short, as the real action was in the operating theatre. We still had individual patients to look after, and occasionally acted as a third assistant, holding a retractor for an hour or so if we were lucky. The registrars and junior residents had priority, needing the experience for their higher surgical degrees. Surgery is not all the excitement depicted by Hollywood or TV, but long periods of time spent carefully exposing and stitching tissues. This meant long periods of boredom, unable to see the action through the backs of the operating staff. We made our own excitement by flirting with the young trainee nurses, whose bright eyes smiled invitingly over their theatre masks, but gave no indication of what the rest of them looked like. We would also visit the other theatre suites where the ear, nose and throat surgeons, or ophthalmologists worked. As they rarely saw students, they were always welcoming and enjoyed explaining the finer points to us. There was never the same degree of tension and the theatre sisters, who usually disliked students getting in the way, were easy-going and pretended to ignore any flashing glances between student and trainee nurse.

We learnt the basics of anaesthesia from an assortment of old and new school anaesthetists. The older ones tended to have red noses and could sometimes be seen sniffing a mask. They were suspicious of new gadgets and were artists in their field, using the older inhalation methods skilfully and remarkably safely. The only monitoring was blood pressure, pulse, the pinkness of the eyelids and degree of dilatation of the pupils which gave an indication of the closeness to death. Their description of anaesthetics was like war, long periods of boredom interspersed with moments of extreme terror. The younger ones used the new pentothal and curare muscle relaxant and had begun to intubate the trachea for safety. These intravenous anaesthetic agents used with gas and oxygen, allowed the surgeon to have a completely relaxed abdomen to operate on, instead of the struggle to work through tightened muscles. It also meant that he could use the electric diathermy without the danger of an ether explosion. The present day anaesthetist's station compares favourably to a jumbo jet's cockpit, electronics continuously recording blood oxygenation, carbon dioxide, pulse rate, blood pressure, respirations, temperature and cardiogram.

We had valuable hour-long sessions in the small teaching room attached to each ward, with physicians and surgeons talking around particular cases. This was when we learnt our most useful medicine, with friendly rivalry setting a high standard of knowledge. Treatment went under the headings of

Regimen (bed or ambulatory), Diet, Drugs, (specific and symptomatic), Bowels and Stimulants, with the bowel action being the ward sister's territory, vigorously enforced by aperient or enema.

The more formal education was by set lectures, covering most subjects, with the more extroverted speakers attracting the largest audiences, regardless of the quality of their material. One retired physician gave an annual talk entitled "Things Are Not What They Seem" to a packed house. His observations were straight out of Sherlock Holmes. He said he could always tell in winter, if the woman who was consulting him had a happy marriage by the blotches on her shins. These were produced by heat from the fireplace, so-called *erythema ab igne*. If they were on one side, she sat sideways opposite her husband and was likely to be happy, and if they were on the front, she sat alone, presumably unhappily. One of his hobbies was to go around the psychiatric hospitals, spotting the small number of depressive patients sitting motionless, requiring feeding, dressing and toileting, who were in reality thyroid deficient. After one month of oral medication, they returned home to the consternation of their families, having slept for years, like Rip van Winkle or Oliver Sachs' encephalitis cases.

I had other occasional and valuable patient contacts outside the atmosphere of the teaching hospital. Some of my group were sent to the Central Middlesex Hospital for a short surgical term when we saw the "bread and butter" cases of hernias and varicose veins, instead of the complex rarities which we had assumed were the norm. I began to realise that most patients would get home in a few days, with their problems cured without undergoing prolonged and painful investigations.

I visited brother Tony at the Brompton Chest Hospital where he was a registrar, dealing particularly with tuberculous cases. Streptomycin had not been discovered and there was no magic bullet to be taken internally. Active tuberculous cavities in the lungs were treated by collapsing the lung to try to obliterate the infected space. This was by the introduction of air into the pleural cavity outside the lung which then shrank under its own elasticity. A primitive apparatus with two glass containers half filled with water which were alternately raised and lowered, pushed a measured amount of air through a three-way tap into the chest. Care had to be taken to get the correct sequence, and Tony told of watching horrified as water instead of air fed into a patient's chest, fortunately without any serious consequences.

For infections of the lower lobe, air was introduced into the abdominal cavity, giving an instant sometimes embarrassingly pregnant look to young ladies, whose disease had already given a flushed and falsely healthy look. Both these procedures were topped up every month or so. Fifteen years later Tony developed early tuberculosis, but quickly settled with antibiotics without having to go through the ordeal of a pneumothorax. TB is a treacherous organism.

In February 1949, when the time came to do our obstetrics course, four of us decided to go to the Rotunda Hospital, in Dublin, for six weeks. The Rotunda had a world wide reputation for excellence, it was an adventure to see another country, the food was unrationed, and the supply of babies abundant and constant. We had to perform twenty deliveries by ourselves, after four under supervision, and in England, there was often competition from student midwives and young doctors, keen to get their quota for their higher qualifications.

The trip over gave us a foretaste of the amiable Irish. Despite the rough seas, the boat from Holyhead to Dún Laoghaire, the port of Dublin, was crowded with farmers and labourers none the worse for the weather, compressed in the bars, drinking Guiness stout, cigarette stubs vibrating on their lower lips as they shouted greetings in delightful, unintelligible accents. At the hospital, we were introduced to the clinical clerk, the obstetrical registrar under whose instructions we were to be prepared to deliver the ladies of the poorer quarters of north Dublin. The attitude of the maternity sisters was different to the cold "get out of my way" demeanour in some of the major London hospitals.

They were warm, welcoming and motherly, always ready to share their knowledge with us, born from an enormous range of deliveries, simple or complicated. We had two Irish students in our two week intake, most of the others being on holiday.

The first baby I saw delivered was by forceps, with an obstructed labour. The clinical clerk sat at the foot of the bed between the stirruped legs of a huge anaesthetised woman, and kept up a cheerful banter with the nursing staff. "Never let yourself get like this," he said, "always stay like this," indicating a particularly petite nurse. When my turn came to deliver a baby, it unexpectedly turned out to be twins. The mother had had no ante-natal visits, which would have revealed her condition. As it was her twelfth pregnancy, she had felt such visits were no longer necessary, despite the increasing danger with "grand multipara" or women with high pregnancy scores. With a lot of noise and shouts of "Be quiet, woman, ye're like a baist in the faild" from the supervising resident doctor, she delivered quickly and easily.

When the time came for us to go out into the district to do home deliveries, the commonest type of arrival in Dublin at that time, the clinical clerk gave us a brief oral examination to assess our range of knowledge and how potentially dangerous we might be to the mothers of north Dublin.

"Now," he said, "any final questions?"

"Yes," said a young Irish student. "What do we do if the waters break?" A look of total disbelief came over our mentor's face.

"Send for the bloody plumber," he whispered.

I was placed on the on-call roster as a junior student, being shown the ropes by a senior student with two weeks more experience. In two weeks, I too, would be classified as senior. We took our bicycles and made our way to Cabra West, a housing estate with a tough reputation. We were instantly recognised as the boys from the Rotunda and were shepherded with tender care to the expectant mother's house. Most of the rough characters had been Rotunda home deliveries themselves and our mission was sacred. A Dickensian figure met us in the hall.

"Thank God you've come, doctor," she said, a huge busy untrained but highly competent midwife in the Sarah Gamp image. "I've got the hot water on and I've been over to borrow the neighbour's razor."

To be called "Doctor" at the age of twenty, with another eighteen months to go to qualify, struck a mixed chord of vanity, pride and not a little apprehension. I could feel my feet of clay and decided to put on a grave, thoughtful and thoroughly professional look, as I joined my senior in the tiny room in which a new Irish soul would first see the light of day. We unpacked the medical bag, which contained the basic obstetrics kit, a bottle of Dettol antiseptic, swabs, pads, sterile string for the cord, scissors, gloves to be boiled up and soaked in Dettol, (this is when I began to get my Dettol allergy).

A primitive mouth-powered suction device like a metal straw with a bulge in the middle was available to clear dangerous mucus from the infant's throat, with two ergometrine tablets in case there was a postpartum bleed. We had no syringes but checked where the nearest telephone box was situated, as any serious complications were dealt with on the spot by the clinical clerk, arriving like the Fifth Cavalry in his little Morris van. He was able to do stitches, forceps deliveries and more heroic procedures, rarely admitting the mother to hospital, such was his expertise and her fortitude. Most of these cases had been seen at ante-natal clinics and were considered good risks, whilst those with potential problems were admitted to the main hospital, where would-be obstetricians from the whole world attended.

We greeted the father and admired his preceding children, and went up to the tiny bedroom, where the mother lay quite contentedly on a simple bed. This was just another labour day to her and she felt totally self-confident, but I had the feeling that she was pleased to see us as a backup for possible problems. We examined her and felt that the baby was in normal position, so we set up our bowls of hot water, spiked with antiseptic, and returned downstairs to chat to the father. Two minutes later,

"Doctor, I think it's coming," and we rushed upstairs in time to catch the little wet bundle as it slid gently onto the bed. "Never trust a Multi," a woman with more than one baby, became a reality. The afterbirth came equally easily and no tablets were needed. Sarah Gamp, who had really delivered the infant, wiped it down, and after a cuddle by the mother, he was placed in an open drawer as a temporary cot. It was when we went downstairs to inform the father of his new son, that the full enormity of the situation struck home. This was the first son after five daughters. Highly delighted, he broached a bottle of Irish whiskey, and poured three full glasses.

"Would ye be after having a drop of the Craitur, doctors?" he beamed. That was my only mistake on that day, but we were soon pointed towards the Rotunda on our bicycles and arrived safely, feeling self-satisfied and rather smug at our performance. It was our duty to visit the family daily to check the temperature and any signs of post-natal complications. The next day, I was greeted at the front door by the mother herself. No comfortable week's rest for her, she had her brood to look after.

Not all the deliveries were so simple. Often, we were called in the middle of the night, and sat around the bed for hours, whilst the labour slowly progressed. Our heads nodded and our eyes would not stay open. Twice, we had to telephone for the Flying Squad, both times when the infant's heart began to show distress, and the labour ended in a forceps delivery, in the bed.

Some of the families lived in appalling conditions. Saint Joseph's Mansions, a gross misnomer, was entered up bleak concrete steps. At one delivery I did there, the father was sitting anxiously outside, whilst the mother lay on old newspapers on an Army great coat covering bare bed springs. A previous baby lay at one end of this bed, and three other small children slept in a cot near the sink. The bitterly cold room had a tiny fire with two small pieces of coal in it, and the one and only chair had had one of its wooden seat slats removed, possibly for fuel. The mother had a past history of tuberculosis and was scarecrow thin. Yet in the whole of that north Dublin district, there was only one maternal death that year, and that was due to another case of advanced tuberculosis. I think the Rotunda lived up to its reputation for excellence in trying circumstances.

After each delivery, we were again on the roster and had little time for a social life. I managed to take one day off in the six weeks, and went to visit Glendalough, an ancient Celtic holy place, two hours out of Dublin. It was set in deep emerald green hills, in misty rain, with a ruined abbey and Celtic crosses beside a still lake, incredibly peaceful. It was just what this young "doctor" needed after many sleepless nights in tiny, uncomfortable rooms, hoping for a successful outcome, and feeling the responsibilities thrust prematurely upon him. We had no medical defence insurance, and the thought of being sued for medical incompetence or mistakes never entered our heads, nor the citizens' of the north Dublin district.

After a midnight delivery, we would cycle back through the empty streets and call in at the Green Rooster, an all-night café, to eat a huge plate of bacon and eggs, delicious and unrationed, while we discussed the birth. Opposite the sleeping quarters, Conway's public house welcomed students, doctors and nurses after a long day's work, in sometimes boisterous fellowship, lubricated with glasses of Guiness stout. There was even a hospital telephone extension direct to the bar. A hospital students' song said it all, sung to the tune of 'There's a Tavern in a Town', ending with:

Bear down, bear down, Mrs. Brown, Mrs. Brown,

I've got two fingers on his crown, on his crown,

And we'll soon have the little bugger out,

Then off to Conways for some stout, for some stout!

I came home to London after the Irish adventure with increased confidence in myself but missed the relaxed atmosphere. The war had just finished, leaving Great Britain in a parlous state, its treasury empty, and its Chancellor of the Exchequer a sombre puritanical man with the motto, "Work or want." No-one in our year was interested in frivolous adventures. London was too drab, and even bread had once been rationed, which had not happened in wartime.

In 1947, my father had been appointed Naval Stores Officer to the Chatham naval dockyard, one of the oldest in England. We lived in a row of twelve terrace houses inside the dockyard premises, which had been built by French prisoners of war in Napoleon's time. They had innumerable rooms for the big families and servants of that time, with eight levels, cellar, basement, ground floor, first, second and third upstairs, attic and flat roof.

Each room had a high ceiling, and the Admiralty fittings were massive with enormous brass door knobs. The back overlooked the dockyard itself, with an incongruous view of submarines in dock behind a row of eighteenth and nineteenth century ships' wooden figure heads, staring defiantly across the river Medway, memorials to the days of sail.

Captain Fletcher was in charge of the large naval hospital nearby, and renewed his Colombo friendship with my father. His daughter Jill and I were nineteen year old students commuting by train to London daily. We introduced ourselves through a carriage window, Jill being identified by wearing homemade rabbit skin gloves. She was studying to become an occupational therapist and was happy to be coached in physiology, anatomy and pathology in the hour's trip into London. We began by comparing notes about our respective boy and girl friends, and eventually decided to cut out these middlemen (and women) and to the secret delight of our parents started a long courtship.

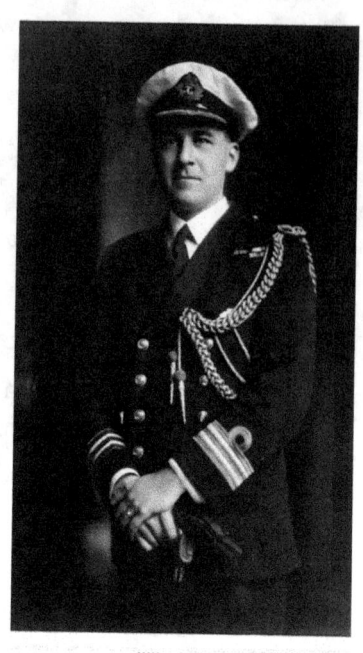

Jill's father
Lt. Cmdr. E.N.R. Fletcher 1931

At weekends, we explored the Kentish countryside on bicycles and spent long hours on the telephone talking nonsense or just listening, not wanting to stop the rapport. On weekdays, we managed to catch the same Chatham train from Cannon St. station in the city, in the same compartment each time, with the other regulars smiling at young love over their Evening Standards, whilst we held hands underneath ours.

After the war had finished. the air shows began. In 1945 at the end of the war, I attended a display of German aircraft at Farnborough, invited by the test pilot brother of a fellow student. There were all the latest types, including many experimental models, a tiny jet fighter, the Heinkel 162 Volksjäger, and a Dornier fighter with an engine and propeller at each end of the fuselage. The disembodied drone of the night bombers we had heard on so many occasions were revealed, and they were demonstrated by low level fly-pasts.

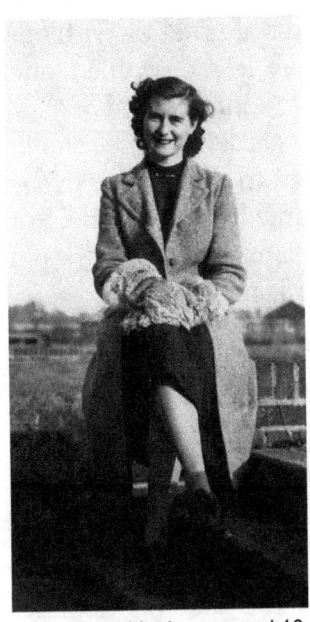

Jill with rabbit gloves, aged 18

Before Farnborough became the venue for the biannual European air shows, the other airfields of Hatfield and Radlett, homes of de Havilland and Handley-Page, were used for displays. As they were all reasonably close to London, I was able to follow the development of the British aircraft industry to its final peak, before the Comet disasters and capitulation to the American giants closed a chapter of aviation history when Britain was still great. I was smuggled into Radlett on one occasion, being given a press pass by a sympathetic departing journalist, and saw Geoffrey de Havilland doing loops from 5000 feet to ground level in the Swallow, a revolutionary tail-less swept wing design in which he was later killed hitting the sound barrier. By 1948, the major annual air show became established at Farnborough, to which I made a pilgrimage as both student and junior doctor. Jill showed her dedication by coming on several occasions.

As the post-war years passed, there was a flurry of other air shows, often presented by a newspaper, and at one of these, I had my first flight, one circuit in a three-seater high wing Auster. Two other private joy flights, both with Jill aboard, completed my early aviating experience apart from major commercial voyages.

Medical students have an unwarranted reputation for wild escapades and debauchery. Every group has its uninhibited members, but so much time is taken up in studying, it leaves little enough for recreation. We had intakes of Oxford University students every three months alternating with our own London University and they were less restrained, and often played harmless, gentle and quite sophisticated pranks. They bulk purchased twenty concrete garden gnomes and in the middle of the night, attached them to every ledge in the six storey hospital, some in quite dangerous positions. For some hours, we had the delightful sight of their little red figures dangling fishing rods over the general public.

In early October each year, the student committee for the Christmas concert was set up. There is always an extraordinary degree of talent in music, song writing and acting to be found in a large teaching hospital amongst the students, nurses and ancillary staff. It is the equivalent of court jesting or Saturnalia, when the shortcomings and foibles of the consultant and administrative staff are held up to gentle ridicule in sketches, songs and pantomime, and they love it. Students were to be seen surreptitiously imitating their walks, mannerisms and speech in preparation for their two minutes on stage. For a consultant to be left out of the concert was a humiliation and we tried to include everyone.

The canteen hall had been cleared of tables and a stage set up at the back. Upstairs, in the biochemistry laboratory which became the changing rooms, the chemicals had been cleared from the benches to make way for wigs, costumes and make-up. A simple screen protected the girls from the boys, or some thought, vice versa. The audience packed in, with standing room only for those who had omitted to get early tickets. We called the show such names as "Foley Bergere" after Foley Street, "Careless Rupture", and "Beau Jest", after our distinguished Dr. Beaumont. (In Sydney, later, the students called one "The Sound of Mucus".) We had three or four main performances, and then toured the wards with selected sketches and songs.

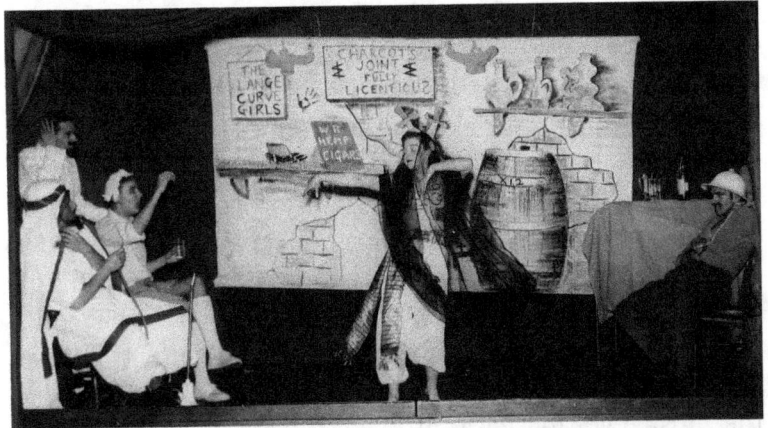

Middlesex Hospital Christmas Concert 1949, featured both Tony and Robin

Every concert had a student impersonation of the nursing staff and my brother Tony was exceptionally good at this, being large and chunky and wearing his pillowed bosom just like some of the battleships who ruled over the wards. He was outstanding, in every way, singing a recruitment rhapsody whilst flinging rose petals out of a bedpan.

Be a nurse, it's such frightful fun.

There's so much to do when the day's work is done.

There's ludo and draughts and walks after dark,
And on Sundays the Girl Guides parade in the park,
And if since an infant, your passion has been
A burning desire for a lavatory cleaner,
Or the carefree, easy life of a char,
Don't hesitate further for here you are,
Join up, join up, be a Nurse.

Despite these distractions, I was able to continue my studies with increased purpose. The final eighteen months was made up of the odd specialities. We attended the gynaecology outpatients and theatre cases, but did not have the personal contact we had had in the main wards. The dermatology ward was a dreadful place, with patients showering dead skin everywhere, and having mediaeval treatment with lotions and baths whose formulary could have come from the Old Testament. Even the consultant seemed to have dandruff. The advent of cortisone and potent antifungal agents has changed the face of dermatology, dragging it into the modern world. The ear, nose and throat surgeon, C.P. Wilson, was an extrovert and very popular for making the most revolting nasal problem interesting. I will always be grateful to him for finally curing Jill's chronic mastoid infection. The ophthalmologist did his best to interest us, but the field was so small for the basics we needed, that a couple of lectures sufficed.

We had several lectures on psychiatry, and visited one of the outlying mental hospitals. The chemistry of the brain was only slightly understood, and there were no psychotropic drugs. Florid cases of paranoid schizophrenia and mania were presented, treated by psychotherapy and sedation, and condemned to a life of wild ideas and occasional padded cells. Psychosurgery, the undercutting of parts of the brain through burr holes, insulin shock and electro-convulsive therapy (ECT) were the active methods of treatment; the former two have fallen into disrepute and the latter has had a renaissance for intractable depression.

Sister-in-law Pat was working as a Sister in a private psychiatric clinic for a short time helping with electro-convulsive therapy. Two electrodes were placed on the head, like earphones and the dose of electricity was dialled on a piece of apparatus similar to the old-fashioned telephone. No anaesthetic nor relaxants were given and the patient went into an acute convulsive epileptic attack, back arched, twitching and eyes rolling. Nowadays, a light anaesthetic and muscle relaxation are used, as the force of the back muscle contracting could cause muscle tears and even compression fractures of the vertebrae. Pat had to ensure that the tongue was not bitten and the airway was maintained, and then to reassure the confused patient on awakening.

This often proved exciting, as the normal social inhibitions had not yet returned. The sight of a very attractive woman bending over male patients sometimes lead to her being chased around the room, to their later embarrassment and contrition.

Jill worked as an occupational therapist for one year at Napsbury, a 2,000 bed psychiatric hospital near St. Albans. Visiting her at weekends had a Dickensian feel, passing through thick doors, opened by a massive bunch of keys carried, chatelaine-like on a large key ring. I glimpsed beds with depression and schizophrenia cases lying curled up motionless. Out in the extensive grounds, manic patients strode about shouting and gesticulating. The main sedation was five to ten mils. of paraldehyde given deeply into the buttock, which sent them to sleep, their breath sickly-sweet, but it was not until Lithium and the phenothiazines like Largactil, that any real control became possible.

The final few months was taken up by the other sub-specialties. We had a small pædiatric ward as most junior patients were sent to Great Ormond Street Hospital, and we had little hands on experience and few lectures. Neurology cases were admitted to a small but interesting ward, interesting because all the cases had physical signs of damaged nervous systems, muscle weakness, loss of sensation or changes to their thinking processes. We learnt to check them from head to toe, the twelve cranial and all the spinal nerves, the eyes for signs of increased pressure or damage to the sympathetic nerves in the neck. We learnt the technique of spinal taps, or lumbar punctures, and followed up the brain tumours in neurosurgery, later to be my first resident post. Regretfully, despite the extensive and enthusiastic documentation, there was no effective treatment for most cases, and there has only recently been improvement, as the brain biochemistry gradually becomes revealed.

During the revision stage before the finals, we sat for hours in the library and looked at the last ten years' examination papers, making educated guesses as to the trend in questions. I had by then become a resident student, living above the resident doctor's quarters, with several students at the same stage. We would revise chapters of textbooks and then sit till late at night, quizzing and counterquizzing, fine-tuning our knowledge. The usual boisterous games of cricket down the corridor became less frequent as one after another buckled down to what we hoped were the final moments of studenthood.

The examinations consisted of several written papers, two each for medicine and surgery, also pathology, pharmacology and obstetrics and gynæcology, but the viva voce and case examinations were the main stumbling blocks which we all feared.

There was no time to think for a couple of minutes. The examiners were right there in front of us. In both surgery and medicine, we first had to examine two "long" cases, being given twenty minutes to take a quick history and make an examination before the examiner returned. My luck held as I had a charming bright eyed young lady who told me the full details about her heart murmur and treatment. There were several "professional patients" who were paid a small stipend to appear regularly for the short cases, when we had to examine a specific organ and talk about the possibilities. The quicker the diagnoses, the more cases were seen in the half hour allotted. We went to teaching hospitals other than our own, but some of the patients' faces were familiar from previous lecture demonstrations. We had a short pathology practical test, identifying twenty slides under the microscope, and talking about specimens in glass pots, which was like looking at old friends, we had studied them so well. Suddenly it was over and I had the few days wait for the results, remembering all the stupidities of my viva exams, certain of failure, for who could possibly pass such crass ignorance. We knew there were numerous ways of being told the bad news at vivas. The gentlest way was for the examiner to go over to the window and look out at the autumn sky and say, "Mr. Jones, it is now approaching winter and all the birds are flying away to warmer lands. But in spring, they will all be back, and so will you, Mr. Jones." At least no-one had said that to me.

On the first of November 1950, the results were posted up outside the University of London, using our examination numbers instead of names. I scanned down for number 150 and found a gap. Martin came up cheerfully. "I got Honours in

Surgery," he said, pointing to a separate list of ten numbers, and there was Number 150, Honours in Pharmacology and Therapeutics, the only subject I thought I had passed. Now came one of those rare occasions in life when there were no responsibilities. The exams had been passed and work as a resident doctor was three weeks away. I had been interviewed and secured the post of neurosurgical houseman. I could offer my fiancée Jill decent long term prospects.[1]

Chapter 4: RESIDENT

I once heard a medical lecturer say that a doctor is three things: technician, witch-doctor and priest. He comes out of medical school a good technical expert in pathology, medicine and surgery, but learns his priesthood in the years of listening to and advising patients, not necessarily on medical matters. And there is still a lot of black magic as suggestion therapy with the old traditional treatments slowly giving way to modern medications whose actions are better understood and more effective, but often with side effects.

In January 1951 I started my life as a doctor, as an over-confident junior Resident to the neurosurgeon at my own alma mater, the Middlesex Hospital, London. My consultant was Miss Diana Beck, the only woman neurosurgeon in a highly competitive male orientated society. She was about forty five at the time, a short, precise, dark haired woman always immaculately dressed in a dark suit. She belonged to the slow school of neurosurgery, that is, she took many hours of meticulous dissection to lay bare a brain tumour, as distinct from the rapid school who felt that even the most intricate of procedures should be accomplished in two hours or less.

She had a senior and a junior Registrar to help in the marathon operating sessions. Often by midday, she would leave to snatch a quick lunch, while the senior Registrar and I picked away through the tiger country of the exposed brain. Then she would continue with the junior Registrar whilst we had our meal. The anaesthetist had organised himself in an ingenious way for these sessions, which could last fourteen or fifteen hours. He sat comfortably outside the operating theatre itself, in a room which housed an electroencephalogram, a large machine used to record the brain's electrical activity. He could watch proceedings through a glass panel, and had hooked up the machine as an electrocardiogram. He could safely monitor the patient, have his cups of coffee and read his newspaper outside the sterile confines of the theatre, entering occasionally to take the blood pressure and change the gas cylinders.

My duties were to oversee the care of twelve neurosurgical cases. These were mostly desperately ill with brain tumours, which we would spend hours exploring, only to retreat with the diagnosis of "inoperable". Occasionally, we had exhilarating moments, when a life threatening blood clot in a head injury from a car accident was removed and the patient awoke from a deep coma on the table, or a malignancy turned out to be noninvasive and completely removable. We also dealt with prolapsed intervertebral discs by excision of the offending disc material, but the results did not seem to me to be very good.

This was in the days before high blood pressure was so effectively treatable. The only medical treatment was a rice diet or extreme sedation by Phenobarbitone or Reserpine, a mysterious Egyptian drug extracted from the root of the Rauwolfia plant, or removal of the lumbar sympathetic nerve chains. The first was a form of salt reduction. To get an appreciable drop in blood pressure, phenobarbitone converted the patient into a zombie.

Reserpine is still used occasionally in pregnancy for hypertension, and lumbar sympathectomy is occasionally used instead of arterial grafting for threatened gangrene of the legs. We performed the latter for very severe life threatening high blood pressure, and although the effects eventually wore off, we had gained time for the advent of more and more effective blood pressure reducers.

Sometimes it was too late. A young woman had presented with increasing blindness, which was found to be due to "malignant hypertension" or very high blood pressure of sudden onset. Both sympathetic chains were removed from the flanks but the pressure plummeted during the anaesthetic. Intravenous drips were in their infancy and tight bandages were applied to all four limbs to try to expand the blood volume to the vital organs, but she never recovered, having been too long without sufficient blood supply to the brain.

The ward was the most depressing in the hospital, and the nursing staff made up for this by being totally committed, accepting the ghastly sight of ex-human beings, lying like vegetables, their brains no longer functioning. The investigations were unpleasant and often very painful. A full neurological examination had to be made of every nervous function of the body as well as the normal physical check of the heart, lungs, abdomen and urine. Spinal fluid was checked by a lumbar puncture, which I did several times daily. This served me well in later days in Nigeria, where spinal anaesthesia was used for most operations below the waist.

Head X-rays show little more than fractures, most tumours being invisible to radiation. Iodine-containing dyes could be injected into the spinal fluid to outline pathology in the spine, but air encephalography was used for defining the contents of the skull. This was an unpleasant procedure, with a small burr hole made in the skull, and a fine blunt needle inserted through a "silent" area of the brain to reach the fluid-filled ventricles, into which air was injected. The density difference between air and brain gave some indication of the underlying pathology, but also one of the worst headaches known, due to the drop in cerebral pressure. For this we gave a mixture of aspirin, phenacetin and heroin, as morphine could depress the respirations and compromise the patient further. What a change from today's technology, when a painless ultrasound, CT scan or MRI shows up all the brain tissues as clearly as wiping the bathroom mirror reveals the morning face in all its glory.

"You don't bother with all that now, doc, you just put their heads in a box," an American doctor friend said. Three dimensional views reveal the extent of tumours and their operability is accurately assessed. Precise radiotherapy can be planned and decisions about chemotherapy made. It was unimaginable in 1951, as no doubt 2051 procedures would be to us now.

Miss Beck was kind to her staff, but would not suffer fools lightly. The brain is too delicate and sensitive to allow mistakes on the operating table. There she became a tartar, and after several hours, became irritable even with her favourite junior Registrar, who suggested privately spiking her morning coffee with a small dose of Phenobarbitone.

On his last day before leaving for another job, he remarked, "How would you like these stitches cut, Miss Beck? Too long or too short?" I think he had already been given his reference.

One problem with that particular residency was the lack of an opposite number for weekends off. All the other wards had two residents and they could take alternate times off, but I was all alone and never had one day off in the whole six months.

Jill, to whom I was then engaged, would come up to the residents' quarters under the watchful but sympathetic eye of the Sister in charge, or we would persuade one of the surgical residents to be on call for a couple of hours while we had dinner (two sausages, chips, tea and as much tomato sauce as we wanted, for one shilling and six pence) at the Glory, a Cypriot café opposite the hospital. We followed by a visit to the pub opposite casualty for a Barley Wine, a thick heavy stout with a punch in it, limited to one only, and a game of snooker in the resident quarters. The pay was £250 per annum less £100 for living in, and I was able to save nearly the whole £75 from my six months salary for our honeymoon in Paris and Austria.

Jill and I were married on 2 June 1951 in Sunningdale church just outside London, from the house where Jill had lived for some time with her cousins, during her mother's illness and father's absence in the Navy. The weather was perfect, my job had finished and we had three weeks all to ourselves. Martin Sawday was my best man and needed a lot of assurance about not dropping the ring. Jill arranged for the Prize Song from the Meistersingers to be played to encourage me while I awaited her arrival. All close family members were present, except Dick and Pat, away in the Sudan. Jill looked the ravishing bride and the speeches were kept to a minimum. We drove away in an old hired Ford Prefect car, and had to return to borrow a key to the boot, in which our luggage had been inadvertently locked. It was a strange sensation to be leaving such a good party which was just starting.

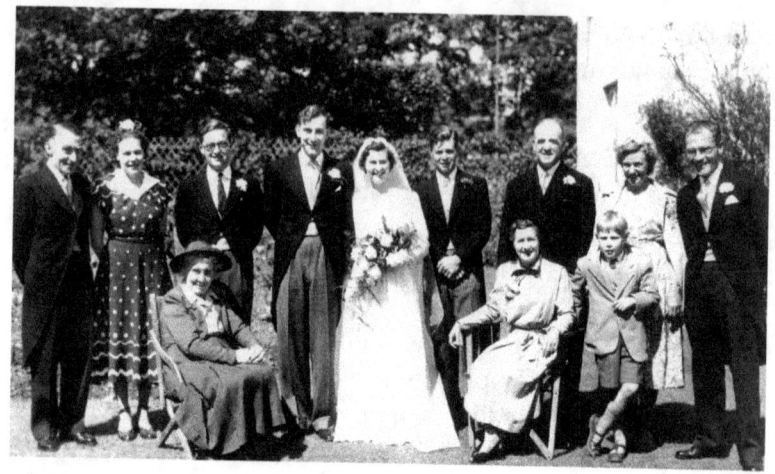

The Wedding.
Front row from left: Grannie Hebb (Robin's grandmother), Kathleen Fletcher (Jill's mother), Adrian (Robin's brother).
Back row: Reginald 'Jelly' (Robin's father), 'Tim' (Robin's stepmother), Bestman Martin Sawday, the groom and bride, Tony Fletcher (Jill's brother), Captain Lyn Fletcher (Jill's father), Joan & Tony Jelliffe (Robin's brother and sister-inlaw.)

Our honeymoon began with a brief flight to Paris, where we stayed at a small hotel near the centre, surrounded by bistros and restaurants. The weather was superb and we walked or used the Metro to be typical tourists, visiting Notre Dame, the Eiffel Tower, Montmartre, the Madelaine, and taking a trip out to Versailles. A bottle of Beaujolais, a metre of crusty bread and assorted cheeses made a heaven on earth for those few days. Paris was still relatively empty, and the Louvre could be examined without the present day schools of tribal visitors, gathered protectively about the guides and their identifying flags. In the hotel bedroom stood a curious little basin, which Jill argued must be for washing tired feet. However it gurgled and glugged all night, and we realised it was a bidet, with a lot of nocturnal activities taking place in adjoining rooms.

We continued the honeymoon by train in a sleeping compartment, but Jill was far too excited to sleep much, seeing the countryside of Europe slip by, and passing through the Customs at the Swiss and Austrian borders in the middle of the night. We left the train at midday at the small town of Landeck, followed by a drive up a narrow winding

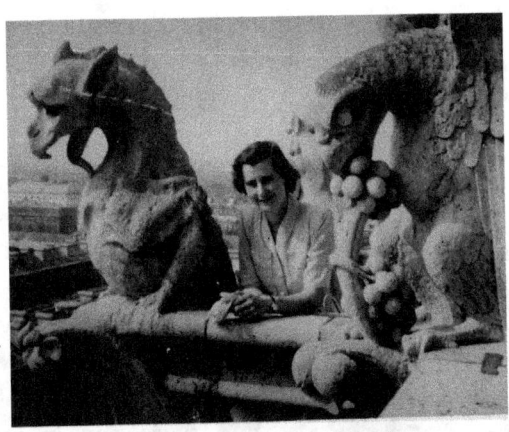

Paris Honeymoon - Jill on Notre-Dame

road, with precipices ready to engulf us, especially terrifying as we drove on what seemed to be the wrong right side of the road. We climbed up towards the snow line, reaching the end of the road at the tiny hamlet of Galtür, where we were welcomed at the Paznauernerhof guest house, as the sole guests in this summer season, presently devoid of skiers.

We spent the days walking over the Tyrolean mountains, through the snow line, managing to get sunburnt, not to be recommended on a honeymoon. There was a small waterfall, the *"schlucht"*, and a *"hohe wanderwege"*, or high wander path, and we quickly learnt that *"zwei bier"* meant two bottles, not glasses, with sufficient schoolboy German to get us understood for the other basic necessities of life. It was here that we were first introduced to the doona and its control on the bed which was vital at the low night temperatures of the high alps.

We flew back to London and Jill stayed with my parents, while I departed south to St. Mary's Hospital, Portsmouth, to take up my next residency. It was very different to the high powered semi-academic world of a teaching hospital. This is where the real bread and butter stuff of medical life presented itself. I had two acute medical wards of ten beds each to share with a Registrar under the care of a consultant physician, and some chronic male and radiotherapy patients. In the female ward, there were several breathless young women with the flushed faces of mitral stenosis. Cardiac surgery was in its infancy. Digitalis in powdered leaf tablets, and injections of mercurial diuretics were the mainstay of treatment. The amount of active substance in the former was assayed by the manufacturer by LD 50, i.e. the "Limes Tod", or death limit of 50% for laboratory rats. Nowadays, precise doses are given in pure form measured accurately by electronics. The mercurial diuretics poisoned the renal tubules sufficiently to leach out large quantities of fluid built up by the cardiac failure, without doing much permanent harm. It was the lesser of two evils. Modern diuretics are safe and can be taken for years by mouth, and heart valves are replaced in plastic or metal, or borrowed from pigs or cadavers, and even repaired.

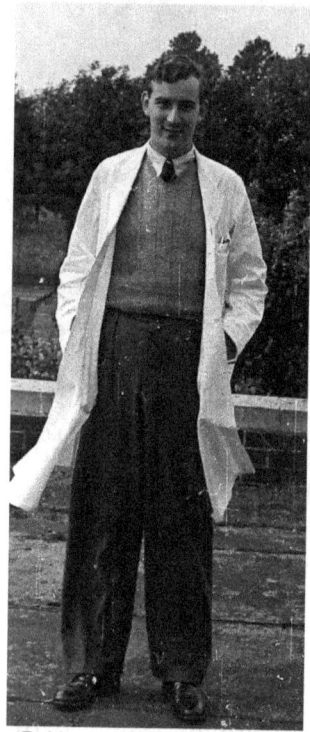

Robin as a Resident Medical Officer at St. Mary's Hospital, Portsmouth, 1951

We ran an outpatient clinic for rheumatoid arthritis, using huge doses of aspirin, and if this failed, weekly injections of gold in a soluble form. It was given empirically as the immune system's workings had not yet been clarified. The only immunity we were taught was that induced by immunisation against tetanus and diphtheria. Many trials of treatment were given without the present day ethical committees to advise and supervise. I wonder why gold was thought of, as it turned out to be very effective in suppressing rheumatoid arthritis and is still an occasional form of treatment.

The cancer patients occupied a small ward and had doses of radiotherapy from machines which lacked the precision of today's high energy apparatus. Chemotherapy was in its infancy. We used nitrogen mustard intravenously. This was a spin-off from observations of the effects of this wartime poisonous liquid on the blood cells. It was highly toxic, and great care had to be used when it was administered through the intravenous drip. Saline was washed through before and after the dose, as any spill into the tissues caused an area of skin to slough. Blood counts were taken daily as the bone marrow and antibacterial activity were depressed. These precautions are taken to this day, but not as frequently, as the range of chemotherapeutic agents has increased and administration is more sophisticated.

Leukemia was a totally fatal disease then, whilst it is now frequently curable. I found an upstairs flat in a road next to Grandfather's and felt strangely at home there, a sort of déjà vu, as the terraced houses were all identical or mirror images. I bought a small 35mm camera and a basic enlarger. Jill and I would spend hours in the kitchen which we converted into a dark room, immersing rolls of black and white film through developing solutions, which gave me an allergic rash on my hands and triggered off a similar response to a chemical in Dettol antiseptic. The six months passed happily and rapidly, although Jill's last month was complicated by vomiting of pregnancy.

After completing my one year's resident posts in 1951, I was to be called up for two years of military service. The prospect of looking at soldiers' feet in a lonely army base off the coast of Scotland did not appeal. With both father and father-in-law well up the ladder in the Navy hierarchy, a posting to her Majesty's ships had been hinted at, but this would have entailed separation from my new bride. There were two alternatives available: a two year tour in Malaya, where a dirty war against Communist insurgents with live ammunition was at its height, or two eighteen month tours in the Colonial Medical Service in Nigeria, still part of the British Raj, where there was a shortage of medical staff.

My brother Dick was senior lecturer in medicine at Ibadan University in Western Nigeria, and I felt he could be a great help, living nearby. I did not appreciate the huge size of the country and when I finally arrived, our posting was six hundred miles away, so I saw him for one day only. We felt that it was an adventure into an exotic country and the chance to see and treat a wide range of diseases, tropical and otherwise, and a valuable experience in self-reliance.

Only one other young doctor took up this offer, and he was posted to the sleeping sickness service in Northern Nigeria, forever on the move between villages, camping out in bush houses. His job was to assess and treat the deadly parasitic disease transmitted by the tse-tse fly, which decimated whole villages in the Savannah belt. The organism attacks the brain, causing a gradual loss of consciousness, and required confirmation by lumbar puncture and prolonged treatment by locally trained nursing staff. He and his wife tired of the constant movement and lack of a proper home, and he preferred to go back to England for military service after one tour.

I had a quick interview and medical examination, and we were both given injections against yellow fever, typhoid, cholera, poliomyelitis, and booster inoculations against smallpox. Jill also had an X-ray to check her pelvic size, as she had recently fallen pregnant. It was not then realised that these could all be potentially harmful to the foetus. Fortunately, our son has never shown any ill effects.

We collected a kit allowance, and attended F.P. Baker's colonial outfitters, the traditional provider of gear for overseas servants of the British Empire. Our basic list to confront the tropics was as follows:

- *Three locked black tin trunks.*
- *Two collapsible camp beds with mosquito netting.*
- *Paraffin Tilley pressure lamps.*
- *Sleeping bags.*
- *Long trousers and dresses with mosquito boots for night time use.*
- *Baggy khaki shorts, long socks and safari jacket and shirts*
- *One tin hip bath with locking lid for both security and hygiene.*

Chapter 5: OUT TO AFRICA

On 7 January 1952, we boarded the MV *Apapa* of 11,000 tons at Liverpool, bound for Lagos. The ship was designed to cross the shallow Lagos bar, and was flat bottomed and consequently rolled in all but calm conditions. Jill had been feeling nauseated with the pregnancy and, we realised later, with the Paludrine anti-malarial tablets which we started one week before departure. Even though the ship was securely tied up at the wharf, she felt worse with the slight motion, and when we went down to the dining saloon, she had to retire to her bunk. For years afterwards, any room with similar stained wooden panelling gave her the same feeling, even on dry land, such was the conditioned reflex

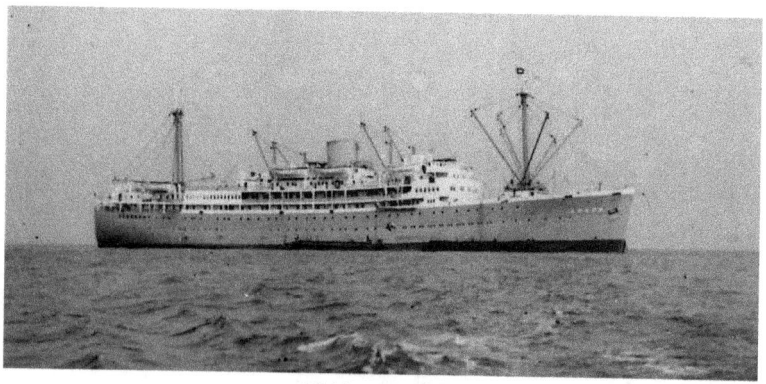

MV Apapa, 1952

she had to fight. The steward reported another passenger down the corridor had an identical problem and passed sympathetic messages back and forth.

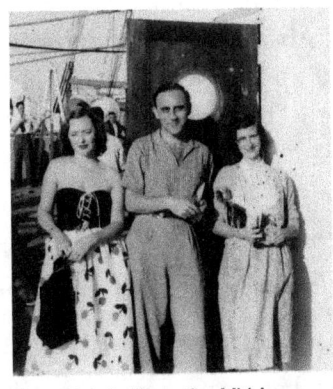

Pat, Dick & Jill on the MV Apapa

By chance, Dick and Pat were also aboard, and we had looked forward to a pleasant fortnight's cruise. The Apapa rolled its way across the storm-ridden wintry Bay of Biscay, and it was not until we passed the Canary Isles that the weather cleared and we enjoyed balmy, sunlit, calm days and clear moonlit nights, ideal for romance under different circumstances. Food became delicious, and the iced water glasses dripped condensed moisture, which was a novel experience for us newcomers, used to British tap water at room temperature.

On gala night, Jill appeared briefly at dinner, to meet her fellow sufferer wearing identical F.P. Baker long dresses, but neither of them really cared. Old Coasters told us tales of the early days in the colonial service, when men were men, and women were not allowed into the country known as the White Man's Grave, before adequate anti-malarials and yellow fever inoculations. One district officer, going to Bauchi in the north, told us of his time in the remote Azare area, regarded as a testing ground or punishment station, full of hardships and lacking any facilities. Duly impressed, we listened respectfully, but felt he must have been exaggerating.

One misty morning, the throb of the engines became muted and we went up on deck to watch the dolphins riding the bow wave and the flying fish gliding across an oily sea, their tail tips vibrating in the surface water. A subtle new odour wafted from the port side, and through the haze, a small outrigger fishing canoe glided past. Half a dozen Africans in it waved nonchalantly, and smoke from a small fire in the stern brought with it the smell of palm oil cooking, as characteristic a smell of West Africa as gum trees were to an Australian homeward bound up the New South Wales coast before the advent of jet travel. The blur on the horizon condensed into a coast line, and the Apapa dropped anchor at Bathurst in the wide mouth of the river Gambia.

Lighters and other small craft came alongside to load and unload cargo and passengers. Dick and I leant over the rail, the old hand and the new boy, observing the exciting scene of brightly dressed women balancing enormous loads on their heads, in graceful upright postures, babies wrapped securely on their backs. Musical shouts and greetings in a tonal language echoed across the foredeck, where they were to sleep for the coastal journey. The men were fit and muscular, but many had bandages around their shins, the curse of the tropical ulcer. One man had a severe dermatological condition, with the skin peeling off his arms, legs and body.

"He'll probably be your cook," said Dick, "and specialise in flaky pastry."

The next port of call was Freetown, Sierra Leone, where we went ashore for a few hours, landing at the old slave steps. The intense moist heat, coming after an English winter, was overpowering. On the boat ferrying us to shore, Jill suddenly said, "I can't see." Pat immediately realised she was about to faint and caught her before she sfell over the side. In pregnancy, one of the main physiological problems is to lose the heat generated by the furnace of the rapidly growing infant, which is why expectant mothers have rosy cheeks and hate summer. Jill could not sweat enough in the high humidity and was overheating. We were driven around the town, every sight new and interesting, small traders with tables laden with colourful merchandise from peppers to dried monkeys, and Syrian, Lebanese and Indian stores. Several cold drinks at a hotel revived us for the boat back to the Apapa, where Jill and I collapsed thankfully on our bunks.

Next port of call was Takoradi, the large artificial harbour in the then Gold Coast, now Ghana, built to allow easier access to the sea along a coast with little natural protection from the Atlantic rollers. In pidgin English, really big is "Plenty big past Takoradi Harbour" and really tasty is "Plenty sweet past kerosene". The harbour was concrete and without the character of a port which had grown into adulthood over centuries of use. I can remember only its bustling activity, and was glad to be on the final stage to Lagos.

We were met at Lagos wharf by an African official from the health department, and, after clearing customs without any problems, were taken to the Bristol Hotel in the middle of town. Our room overlooked the main street, and the sounds of street traders and traffic kept us awake most of the night. It was a dark, dank room, and the mattress, sheets and pillows smelt of sweat. There were no mosquito nets, as we were told that there were no mosquitoes in the middle of town. I proved them wrong by getting a badly infected upper eyelid from a bite, which needed penicillin and kept me longer than expected in Lagos.

I visited the medical hierarchy and was told to get a car, with a loan which was payable back over five years, the exact amount of the monthly car allowance, a way of ensuring that I looked after the vehicle. I decided on a Standard Vanguard Estate, which was serviced by a Swiss company, UTC and had a good reputation for bush work. The medical administrative officer in charge was unsure of our final destination, and was

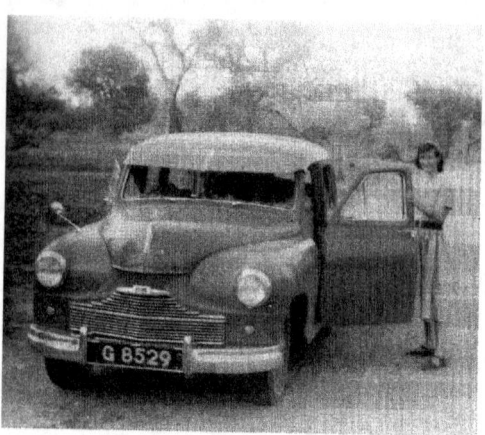

Jill with standard Vanguard

horrified about our hotel. We had one more night there, lying on our coats on the grubby beds. In the middle of the night, Jill said a mouse had scuttled across her, but we found it to be a large cockroach.

The next day, we moved to the Government Rest House complex at Ikoyi, out of the town centre amidst luxuriant tropical gardens, our first contact with hibiscus and bougainvillea. The cabin was spotlessly clean and mosquito-proofed. The dining room provided curries or ground nut stew, with over twenty little side dishes of mangoes, papayas, coconut, banana, cucumber, onions and peppers. After two terrible nights when I had wondered what I had let Jill in for, we had a wonderful sleep.

I went to the garage and completed the purchase of the car, blue with red upholstery, while Jill went to open an account at Kingsway stores, as we had to rely on mail order goods of all kinds. These were transported by train and truck to our destination, often with a six weeks delivery delay. We christened the car with a drive to Victoria beach and watched the fishermen bargaining for their catch with the local women, against a background of palm trees leaning steeply out over the Atlantic ocean.

Back in Ikoyi, we met more Old Coasters and listened to their often outrageous tales of adversities and triumphs over a harsh land. The next day, I was told that we were posted to somewhere in the Northern region, destination still uncertain.

I was to drive eight hundred miles north to the regional capital, Kaduna. We loaded up the car with as much luggage as was mechanically safe, and set off on the main road to Ibadan, to stay overnight with Dick and Pat. We drove slowly and carefully, mindful of the habits of the local population in fatal accidents, which was to dispatch the driver too. There were many large timber trucks occupying the centre of the road, and mammy wagons, transporting goods with a surface coating of people clinging to every possible vantage point, all potentially catastrophic accidents in the making. Every few miles, a cannibalised wrecked truck chassis confirmed my opinion that driving in Nigeria was not to be taken lightly.

On arrival, Dick and Pat showed us the extensive and beautifully laid out University campus, and the five hundred bed hospital under construction. Ibadan, even in 1952 occupied a sizable area, with half a million people, the largest true African city, not counting Cairo, and fifty-five years later, must now be a megalopolis of frightening proportions and problems.

After getting the car serviced, we set off north and ran out of bitumen road after fifty miles, coming onto the laterite surface which made up the majority of all the country roads. This is a red dirt, high in iron content, which is a good wearing surface, but has the unfortunate characteristic of forming corrugations about six inches apart, which become deeper with the passage of time and traffic. The result in a well used road can be bone juddering, and a speed of over 50 mph is necessary to ride on top of the ridges. At corners, the corrugations expanded both in depth and width ensuring a bone-rattling sharp turn, during which I could feel the pound notes peeling off my new car. The red laterite dust billowed out behind us, and a fine layer was sucked in through the vertical back doors, gradually coating all our luggage and finally ourselves with a Santa Claus effect.

We reached Ilorin by 5 p.m. after 100 miles, and booked into a clean government rest-house, glad to shower off our red veneer and to have stopped vibrating, suspecting that this mode of travel would be ours for the next eighteen months. We met more Old Coasters full of information about tomorrow's journey and the Niger river we had to cross.

In the morning, after taking two hours to drive 70 miles on an atrocious road, we arrived at Jebba on the banks of the mighty Niger river. Fortunately we were in the middle of the dry season as in the wet season it can be five miles across in places. The Niger has two separate high water times, one from the local rains, and one from the rainy season many hundreds of miles to the west in Senegal. It had one long bridge at Jebba, designed for the railway, but letting vehicles through along the tracks. Nervously, we ran up onto the line and drove over slowly, dedub, dedub, dedub, trusting that any oncoming trains were, if not on schedule, at least late, but not so late as to be yesterday's.

Thirteen miles further on, we crossed another small tributary, in a much more romantic style, poled across on a pontoon. A further hundred miles of corrugations took us to Bida, where we repeated the process of washing off the laterite dust, having a series of long drinks, meeting colonial officers, and getting gratefully into bed under the mosquito nets.

Jill went through her standard pregnancy breakfast ritual of craving for a kipper, and rejecting it down the toilet, or into a drain, if the nausea was too urgent. By this time, she had managed to keep most meals down, and we set off again in good spirits, well hydrated for the hot, dry journey. The countryside's character was slowly changing from the rolling plains of the Middle Belt, to the Central Plateau of old volcanic rocks. There were numerous villages with straw-roofed mud huts, the villagers coming out and waving. Our car must have been a welcome diversion for them in an otherwise dull day for we passed no other cars for miles on end, apart from an occasional mammy wagon careering dangerously in the middle of the road. Groups of huge smooth grey boulders, like miniature mountain ranges, stood on each side the road, with more huts, goats, donkeys and waving people as we neared the large and ancient town of Zaria.

We had taken over seven hours to cover 270 miles, and repeated our routine of bath, dinner, Old Coaster talk, and welcome bed. For the first time, we needed blankets, as we had left the coastal humidity and reached the continental inland winter climate of warm days and cool nights, which Jill really appreciated.

It was only a short fifty mile drive on the bliss of a properly made up bitumen road to Kaduna, the administrative capital of the Northern Region, set down in territory not affiliated with any particular tribal group. This was on the same principal as Canberra was set down in open Australian bush as an independent capital territory. The roads were wide and well kept, with imposing buildings, housing the Parliament, government offices and the senior officials' residences, with established gardens of tropical flowers and shrubs, which we had not seen since Ibadan. It was obviously a show case on which money had been spent lavishly, much like Canberra.

I introduced myself to the Regional Director, who had wondered where I had got to, there being a breakdown in communication with Lagos. He had no concrete plans, but asked me to go to Azare, the hardship station we had heard about on the Apapa, to relieve the African doctor who needed treatment for an amoebic liver abscess, just for a few weeks. "We won't forget you," he promised, and thought I would then be sent for three weeks relieving at Bauchi, a pleasant town on a plateau near Jos, at a reasonably high cool altitude, then possibly as a field officer at Jos or Gombe, another Azare-like town. The possibility of moving around so much with either a very pregnant wife or a newborn infant was worrying.

The next obstacle was to hire a cook-steward, as it is virtually impossible in the smaller towns for a wife to cope with household duties, going to market for fresh supplies and cooking over a rather primitive wood stove. We chose Sule Jalingo, a stocky young man of the Hausa tribe, since that was the majority language group of our region. His face had been scarred in his traditional markings, the cheeks and forehead ridged with thickened keloids, induced by rubbing ash into fine incisions made in infancy. His salary was £3.15s a month. Mine was £57 a month.

Alas, we had not made a good choice. He became more and more insolent and disorganised. Our stores mysteriously dwindled despite being locked away. To Jill, used to the high efficiency inherited from her Naval father, and her previous occupational therapist's training, he became a severe irritation. The final straws were the washing of the floor brush in the washing up water before the dishes, and the ultimate destruction of all our wedding present glass Pyrex dishes, by being placed directly into cold water whilst still oven hot, despite many warnings and explanations. We realised that there is much to be read between the lines of cooks' references, the classical one being, "This cook leaves us for reasons of health. Ours." Sule was the first of a series of such servants.

Our final 170 miles to Jos was through the fantastic wonderland scenery of an old volcanic plateau. We climbed to 4000 feet amidst scenes such as we imagined the moon's surface to be like, impressions confirmed many years later when the first moon landing was made. The villages are completely different from the Zaria area. They are mostly inhabited by simple pagan tribes who subsist by farming sorghum, millet and maize, with goats and a few Zebu humped cattle for milk and protein. Their huts are made with corn stalks, set amongst the smaller rocks, and they wear very little clothing.

Each of the many small tribes has a different distinguishing style of skirt, which would indicate the women's marital status and number of children, according to the position and number of rings or pieces of grass around their midriffs. Each tribe has its own language and often these bear no resemblance to any others. As we neared Jos, we passed more and more of the local people, sometimes with incongruous articles of clothing, tennis shoes and little else, and then the more sophisticated southerners working for the tin mines of the Jos plateau.

Due to a misunderstanding, our bookings for the Hill Station had not been made, and it was suggested that we use the Army Leave Station instead. This proved to be an excellent, clean and delightful group of whitewashed circular huts with thatched roofs, and separate washing facilities, better than an English holiday camp. We met the Senior Medical Officer, Dr. Campion (who was later to deliver our first born) and the nursing sisters, and loaded up the car with provisions.

The eastern road leaving Jos runs for several miles over rolling bare hills, before a steep gradient downward at Panshanu Pass. A group of baboons sat on the rocks

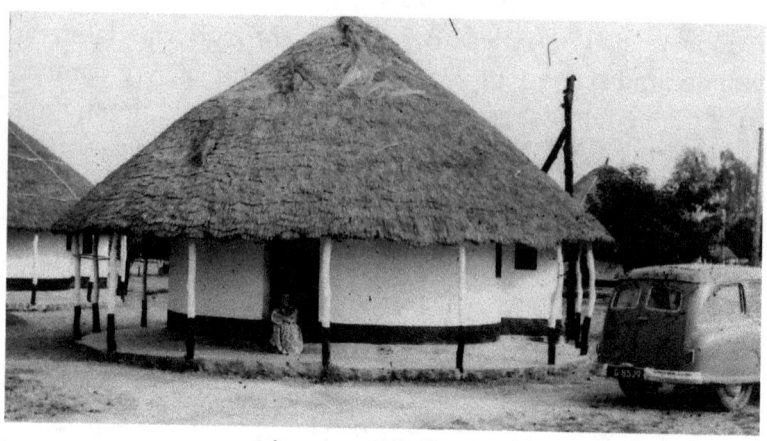
Army Leave Station, Jos

overlooking the road, making what in human terms would have been crude, threatening gestures. As we left the higher country, we saw an increasing number of animals, camels loosely hobbled at the front legs, a wretched muzzled hyena led by an African on a long piece of rope, and the common bird of the high savannah, the hornbill.

Stopping for a cup of tea, a nest of bull ants reminded us that Africa has wild life not to be trifled with. Little processions of donkeys, overloaded with panniers of agricultural produce or huge bundles of guinea corn stalks were guided by Africans, their feet retracted to avoid ground contact, astride the leading animals. The inevitable mammy wagon thundered dangerously past, raising clouds of red laterite dust, masking any vision of other traffic. Worse was the mammy wagon ahead, still in the centre of the road, unable to see us behind, with the dust blocking the sight of oncoming vehicles. It is small wonder that terrible accidents are so common.

In Bauchi, we introduced ourselves to the Medical and District Officers, before setting off for the final one hundred and forty miles to a small town called Potiskum, on the road to Lake Chad. This was the nearest place to Azare where we could get accommodation such as it was, a very dirty rest house with unappetising food, and a District Officer, near the end of his two year tour, who was both unhelpful and pessimistic about our chances of ever seeing our luggage again. His pessimism was contagious, and we left early in the morning for Azare. There were not even any kippers for Jill's morning routine.

We passed long camel trains, ridden by menacing figures completely swathed in dark blue, with swords at their sides. We later found these were very pleasant tribesmen, Buzus, from the southern Sahara, who paid their taxes by carting slabs of salt from ancient pans in the desert, slung on the camels' sides. They made excellent night watchmen, as they were difficult to see in the dark, silent as mice and had a fearsome reputation with their swords.

The hamlets became more numerous, each with a wall of guinea corn stalks. As it was the dry season, goats roamed about freely, picking up whatever they could find amongst the stubble in the dry, harvested fields. More and more of the houses were made of mud brick with the corners of the roofs pricked up into little ears, and prosperous villagers waved us along. At last, we saw a township ahead and passed through the gateway into Azare town, which was to be our base for the next eighteen months.

We met the District Officer, Waller Wood and his wife Jean, had a quick look around the town, dumping the car luggage in his garage. We had to return to stay at Bauchi for seven more days until our main luggage arrived in Azare. They were not spent in vain, as we met our counterparts and district officers, and absorbed a lot more folk lore and tips on how to manage in the remote bush areas.

A violent electrical storm hit on the sixth evening and it rained all night with spectacular sound effects. The next day,

Sule came up and said "Kingi he dead. Me sorry", so we now had Queen Elizabeth the Second. This held us up further as all the government offices closed in mourning.

On our last day, three Americans, one very bouncy and garrulous, from the Sudan Interior Mission turned up in their little Cessna aircraft. At lunch they bent their heads to give thanks which went, "Lord we thank Thee for this food and who is this young lady," looking at Jill, in one continuous sentence. We saw them off at the airstrip, after they had looked inside the engine cowling and fixed something with a piece of wire. Their faith was justified, as they lifted off across the hills with a steady engine beat.

Our final acquisition was Monday Moman Waja, an adult "small boy" to help Sule, at ten shillings a week. Thus fully equipped, we finally set off for Azare.

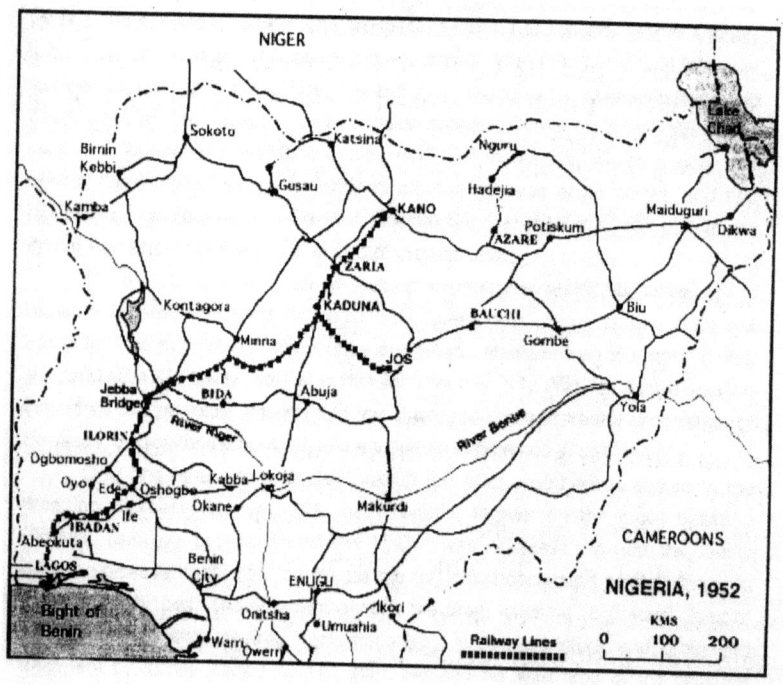

Chapter 6: AZARE

Like most of the towns and cities of northern Nigeria, an Emir at the head of a Native Authority controlled the destinies of the local population. Through them, the British who were then ostensibly in charge, dealt with legal matters, development, and public works. No expatriate was allowed to own land and settle so there were no land claims nor unpleasantness such as occurred later in Kenya and Zimbabwe. The whole annexation of the area seemed to have been by sheer chance, backed up by the apprehension of the numerous imperial European powers at the turn of the century that their rivals would acquire a larger slice of Africa first.

In 1902, a small contingent of soldiers had been sent to punish a group of villagers who had objected to some missionaries. A simple strategem, the segregation of the womenfolk, soon persuaded the tribesmen to sue for peace, as they missed their home cooking and home comforts. The soldiers pushed on to Kano, the major city of the sub-Sahara, fired their field gun at the city walls, and accepted the friendship of a population who could clearly see the advantages of trade and the disadvantages of conflict. The principle of indirect rule through the Native Authority continued with the Nigerians getting a good bargain and a peaceful few decades. There was a saying that, under the British, "A virgin could walk from Sokoto to Birnin Kebi with a basket of eggs on her head, and neither would be spoiled".

My first official visit was to the Emir of Azare, who was dressed in flowing white robes and head dress, and lived in a collection of cool mud buildings in the middle of the town. My Hausa language textbook told me that it was polite to murmur "mm, mm" during a dialogue, just as we say "uh-huh" in English, and I nodded wisely as though I understood everything. It made me determined to learn Hausa sufficiently well to hold intelligent conversations on most subjects.

The sixty-bed Azare hospital serviced about three hundred thousand people, and an area the size of Wales. It consisted of one concrete block male ward, and several other smaller buildings for the operating theatre, outpatients and dispensary. A mud wall surrounded a separate female ward, and I was the only male allowed inside, due to the strict Moslem tradition of purdah. However, the wearing of veils was not practised and the women liked to show off their facial tattoos which were much more decorative and finer

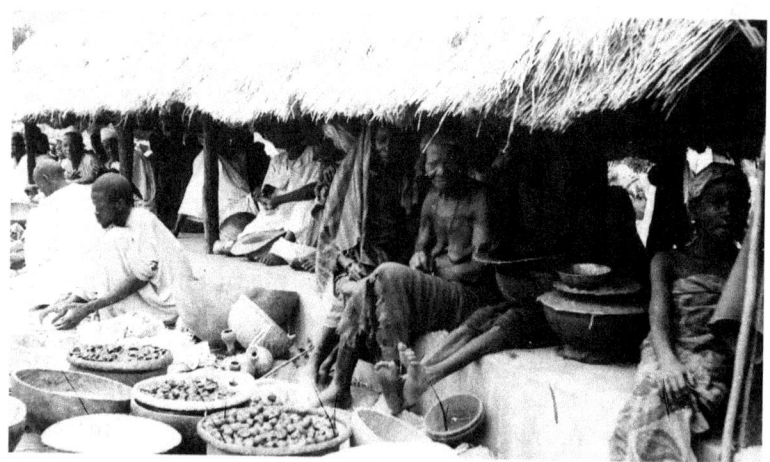

Market scene near Azare, 1952

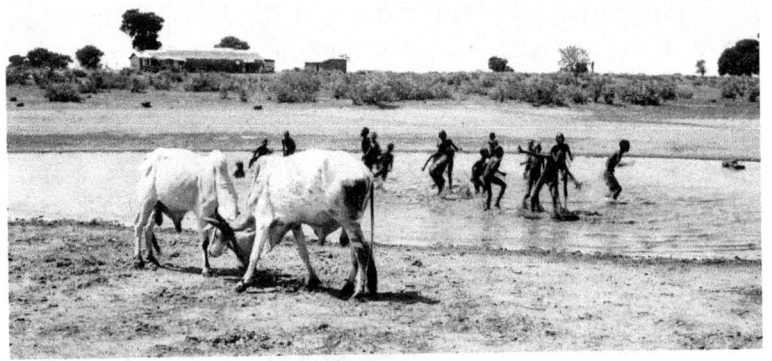

Bulls and children in seasonal fadima, near Doctor's house, Azare, 1952

that the mens'. The senior male nurse was a Yoruba from the Ilorin area of the south-west, and the senior female nurse was an Ibo from the Eastern region. All the other staff were locals, and one of my duties was to train them.

My chief clerk was Mallam Bello, *Mallam* being the title for an educated person. He was a quiet man of about thirty, very polite and anxious to please. He was the most conscientious person I met in Northern Nigeria, where an easy going fatalistic attitude was normal. Mallam Bello paid for it by developing a duodenal ulcer from anxiety. I operated on him for this, two years later in Kano.

My chief outpatient nurse was Mallam Adamu, a man of my own age, twenty-four, whom I soon regarded as a friend and not a subordinate. We were able to talk about many subjects openly, including racial differences from the African point of view, which most white officials were too reserved to discuss. He said white people had an acid smell and was disgusted when he tried a Danish Blue cheese sandwich, telling me it was rotten. He acted as my interpreter, as he had a fair knowledge of English and basic medicine.

I quickly learnt simple Hausa, for it was obvious that Mallam Adamu translated only what he thought I needed to hear. Fortunately, Hausa is a relatively straight forward language, without the tonal modulation of the Yoruba and Ibo, which allows messages to be sent over long distances by intonation of their drum beats and makes hilarious listening for them when an inexperienced white man (or Baturi, meaning red man) attempts conversation. There are only four slight pronunciation differences in Hausa from English. The "A" can be long or short, and the "G", "B" and "D" can be implosive or shortened. Nouns and verbs can be interchanged by simple suffixes and there are a number of words of Arabic origin such as the week days, *"Lit'nin, Talata, Laraba, Alhamis, Juma'a, Asaba, Lahadi"*. A few English words have crept in, "Doctor" becomes *"Likita"* and "Hospital" is *"Asibiti"*.

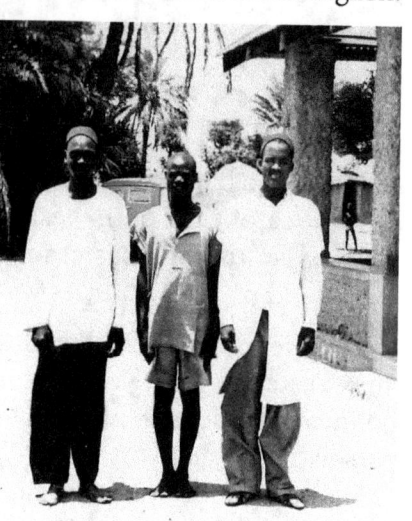

Mallams Bello and Adamu

Mallams Adamu and Bello became my teachers and I was soon able to hold basic medical conversations, usually about the place and duration of the patient's pain or if they had the scourge of syphilis, as distinct from gonorrhoea, which was just a sign of puberty. My mornings began at 7.30 a.m. before the sun became too fierce, seeing up to thirty outpatients by 9.30 a.m. before I drove the two miles back to my house for breakfast.

There I pored over a surgery book propped up on the teapot to see how I was to do the next surgical procedure. I then worked from 10 a.m. to 2 p.m., either on the wards or in the operating theatre, before returning home to sweat out the baking hot afternoon, then back for a final hospital round at 4.30.p.m. At 6 p.m., the sun dropped with disconcerting speed without the benefit of twilight, triggering crescendo after crescendo of massed frog calls from the shallow seasonal lakes in the wet season.

There are only two recognisable seasons in the sub-Saharan region, the wet and the dry. At Azare's latitude, the dry season lasted nine months. As the rains stopped, the days became cooler and quite pleasant and by the northern winter, the Harmattan arrived, a fine dust blown down from the Sahara which covered the tables and windows, causing intense static electricity. We needed a blanket at night, which threw off crackles of sparks. I saw the cat bend down to lap its milk and jump back as a spark earthed its tongue. Touching the car door handle gave an unpleasant little jolt and even a friendly marital kiss was mildly hazardous, although we laughed it off as the spark of true love.

It became one of the driest places on earth. The wooden dining table shrank leaving a half inch gap down the centre, whilst the window frames let in the dust. The wet season took about one month to mature into actual rain. The

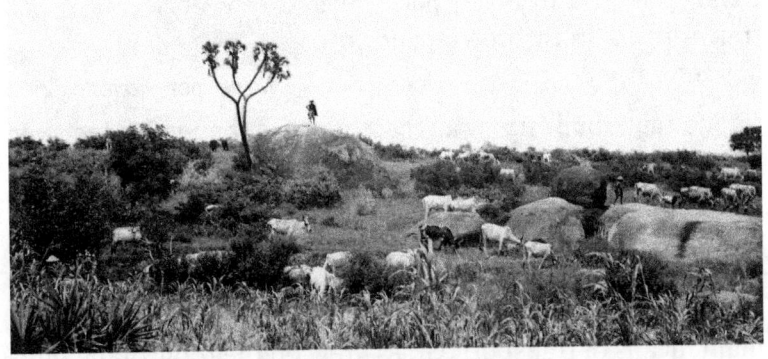

Fulani cattle, near Azare, 1953

relative coolness of the dry slowly gave way to increasing heat and humidity as the moist coastal air moved inland six hundred miles northwards. Storm clouds gathered at night, dissipating at first, but later swirling into huge violent dust storms with continual flashes of lightning and crackling thunder.

Our house was built on a ridge which must have had a base of ironstone. The lightning conductor, a piece of thick bare copper outside the window, twanged and vibrated as it took the charges from the roof to earth. The parched ground outside glowed and flickered through the dust like an early cinema film with full sound effects. After an hour of histrionics, peace returned and with it, the stifling heat and humidity until the next evening performance.

We began to notice the exciting moist earthy smell of rain, days before it finally fell. One evening, the welcome sound of large rain drops on the roof heralded a short downpour, but it was a temporary relief, cooling us but increasing the humidity further. Within two days, the countryside had been transformed from brown sand into a green carpet.

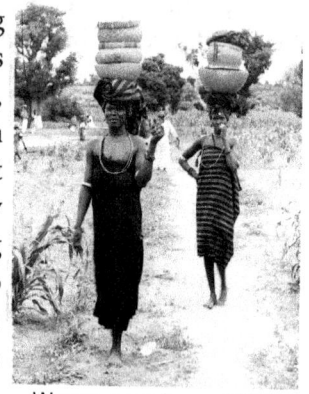

Women near Azare, 1952

The rains built up to a crescendo and then subsided over a three month period. The farmers had planted their staple crops of maize, sorghum and millet, and fenced off their goats, which had scavenged widely for food in the dry season. The side roads became impassable to motor traffic as the dry river beds filled up, and the horse and donkey became the main means of transport. Grass grew on the roofs of the mud houses, mould appeared on clothing and shoes, and wild life, principally insects, but also gazelle, arrived to feast on the greenery. The days of heat and headaches were over for the year. Smallpox and meningitis gave way to malaria.

Our house was built of concrete blocks, designed for the coastal region and totally unsuitable for the baking hot sub-Sahara. The other two government officers had more traditional mud-brick houses with thatched roofs, far cooler, but with a tendency for scorpions and other creatures to drop out at inconvenient moments. Our house was newly built and stood on a bare sandy ridge, with no vegetation or shade trees to mitigate the glare. There was no flyscreening and we slept under hot mosquito nets. Jill felt the heat badly in her pregnant state, as the cooler weather gave way to the build up of humidity before the rains.

Waller Wood, our District Officer, realised her plight and had the bare corrugated iron roof covered with thatch, and organised an outside extension for sleeping, covered with mosquito-proof wire. This was put up by a working party of prisoners from the gaol, in the charge of a "trusty", identified by a sash across his chest. They were a happy joking group, with a series of tricks, such as putting a scorpion perfectly safely on their heads, under their hats, which they removed respectfully, laughing uproariously at our surprise. None of them ever attempted to escape as they would have been chased by their fellows, and anyway, a month or so in gaol was not considered a great hardship with good food, reasonable shelter, and judging by the incidence of acute gonorrhoea, the local girls were allowed in at night.

We had no electricity, and relied on a kerosene fridge for cooling the drinks. Every evening, Sule had the ceremony of lighting the kerosene lamps, usually managing to smoke the inside of the glass. In the season before the rains, waves of different types of insects hatched and become a plague around the lamps, which we stood in bowls of water, to catch them as they plunged down with singed wings. Around the edge and under the fridge, attracted by the small flame, a group of opportunistic frogs and sometimes a scorpion waited to pounce on stragglers.

One extraordinarily voracious type of beetle armed with two sets of jaws, acting both sideways and vertically, was called *"Dokin kunama,"* or the scorpion's horse. It was the fastest thing on six legs and if placed in a jar with a beetle, demolished it as quickly as any prehistoric velociraptor out of a dinosaur movie.

Our worst insect enemies were the stink bugs, tiny shield beetles a quarter of an inch long which swarmed in their millions in the buildup to the rains. They did not sting or bite, but gave off a sickly smell on being squashed, which happened persistently on closing drawers, doors and windows, putting keys in locks and just being stepped on. They were resistant to all chemicals and enjoyed D.D.T., acid, or alkali. In the daytime, they lived between the roof and the ceiling, crawling down at night to drop into the food and other suicidal positions where we were sure to squash them. The only way to lighten the stink bug load was to go up between the roof and ceiling, and sweep them into five gallon tins and then cremate them with kerosene.

For a short time, we had to take great care not to swat a pretty dark green bug if it landed on us. This was the cantharides beetle, which exuded an exceedingly irritant fluid from its joints which caused a chemical burn which took weeks to heal. It has been used in the past as a dangerous aphrodisiac.

We had no telephone, not even from the hospital to the house. Perhaps this was an advantage, as all messages were conveyed by bicycle, and the staff reserved this journey for really important problems. Every Wednesday, a truck brought the mail 140 miles from Bauchi with news from England. We then had a frantic evening, writing replies both personal and official, to catch the Thursday outbound mail. On Saturdays, telegrams and very urgent mail were brought by a man on a bicycle, armed with a bow and arrow against robbers. We heard news of the outside world by short wave radio at night, but our main evening's entertainment was to listen to music on the District Officer's wind up gramophone. "Call me Madam" was my favourite record which still conjures up the cool of evening, the deafening frog calls from the *"fadima"*, a seasonal shallow lake, and the distant drumming from Azare town.

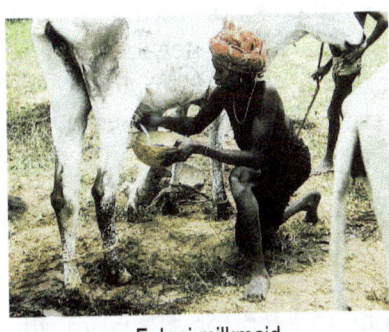
Fulani milkmaid

The garden boy pulled our water up from our well in a goat's skin bucket. He tipped it into a 44 gallon drum for our bath, after heating in a kerosene tin. It was also boiled and filtered for drinking. Itinerant Fulani herdsmen filled a clean empty beer bottle, left in a pre-arranged place and plugged with a twist of grass, with fresh milk from their Zebu cattle herds. A common practice was to adulterate it with dried powder from the baobab tree's fruit. The milk was then boiled, and the fat skimmed off so that Jill could spend a quarter of an hour shaking several day's accumulation to make a reasonable form of butter.

The basic toileting arrangement was called the B.G. for *"Bayan Gida"* meaning the back of the house in Hausa. A simple "thunder box" had a seat over a large can which had a little sand in the bottom. A little more sand was trickled over the contents after use and the whole can was removed daily through a small back door. We asked the Serakin or chief of the *Bayan Gida* to knock before so doing, to reduce embarrassment and to prevent the user being suddenly suspended over an empty space. He always greeted us by bending one knee with a straight back and the can, empty or full, balanced on his head. A new district officer called Backhouse caused considerable local amusement.

Fresh food was limited. Sule went to the market for eggs, of which there were three main types: "market hegg, garden hegg and hegg fit for scramble only". Meat came fresh from the slaughter slab, after examination by the health inspector, whose reports frequently stated "pimply guts", which could have been anything from tuberculosis to worms. It was usually very tough with a gritty taste, and needed a lot of cooking to protect us from infection. Later in Ibadan to tenderise it, we wrapped it in crushed papaya leaves.

Salads and uncooked vegetables were forbidden, being a source of intestinal parasites. We grew small bitter tomatoes in our front garden, sustained by bath water during the long dry season. Sule and subsequent cooks bought live ducks and chickens the size of pigeons to keep for special meals, but a surprising number "done go for bush", in reality into Sule's own cooking pot.

Occasionally, I would go hunting guinea fowl which were abundant around the nearby dried up river bed . I would creep up as silently as possible, rifle at the ready, but they had seen me long before and kept exactly the safe distance away, so very few reached the cook pot. At the end of the wet season the *"fadimas"* filled with ducks and geese, one type being the black spurwing, with a five foot wing span. I was very shaken on one hunting trip, when about to fire at a cluster of geese on the water three hundred yards away, when they all arose in the shape of small children having a bathe. Another occasion, I had hit a duck which was still twitching, so I upended my .22 rifle and dispatched it with a blow to the head. Jill later asked me what the second shot was, and I realised I had reloaded and the gun had gone off over my shoulder. Ten years later in Australia, I operated on a man who had done the same with a snake, but had been hit in the stomach.

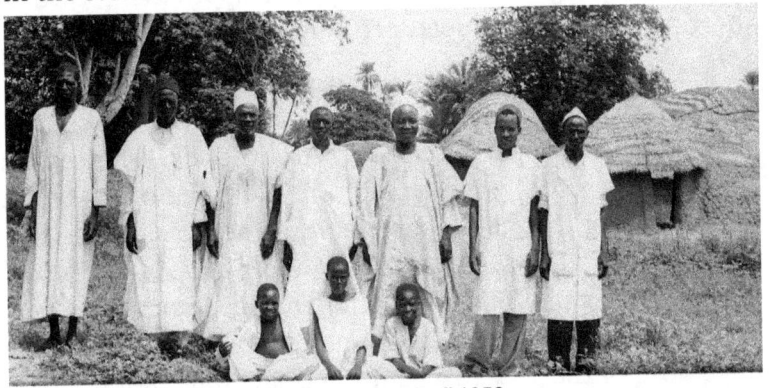

Azare Hospital Staff 1952

These were rare expeditions, most of my time being taken up by the hospital work. The outpatients' room was spartanly equipped with a table and chair for the doctor, a jug and basin of water for washing, a mobile screen, a couch and little else. A queue of male patients stood half way through the door and out onto the balcony. Sexually transmitted diseases were the commonest conditions seen and reflected the open attitude to sex.

Men called it woman's disease, and women called it men's disease. During one year, I saw over a thousand fresh gonorrhoea cases, and eight hundred syphilis cases in every stage from the acute genital ulcer to an aneurysm pounding its way through the breast bone. I had no laboratory tests and the diagnoses were visibly obvious.

The treatment for gonorrhoea was one injection of precious penicillin, while syphilis cases were given intravenous N.A.B., an arsenical preparation. This was very popular as a supposed aphrodisiac. The reasoning went thus: "I have a painful genital ulcer and I cannot sleep with my women. The yellow injection cures my ulcer. Therefore, even if I do not have syphilis, having an intravenous injection will improve my sexual performance". I was often approached with a knowing look, "I want doctor to help me with an injection".

In the outlying towns, the dispensary attendants, the equivalent of the Chinese bare-foot doctor, gave out simple medicines and applied dressings to wounds. They were allowed to give only one type of injection, the other heavy metal used for the plague of syphilis, namely bismuth in the form of bismuth oxychloride. They were under the control of the local Emirs, one of whom demanded and was given weekly injections for his failing potency. He accumulated a huge dose of the very toxic substance and much of his skin peeled off.

My budget for the hospital's drugs and dressings was tiny, and totally inadequate for the number of patients seen. Penicillin was dearer than N.A.B., hence the continued use of this toxic substance. Used procaine penicillin bottles often found their way to the black market, and were refilled with condensed milk and bought by gonorrhoea sufferers for injections by enterprising unqualified entrepreneurs. The foreign protein reaction caused a very high temperature which may have helped destroy the bacteria.

A common complication of gonorrhoea was gonococcal arthritis, very resistant to antibiotics, but which responded well to very high body temperatures. Often, they would self-cure with a malarial fever, but otherwise, we gave intravenous typhoid vaccine which induced a severe pyrexia, standing by to cool them off if their temperature stayed too high for too long. After a lecture to the male nurses on sexually transmitted diseases, I asked them how to avoid contracting them. "I would be very careful whom I sleep with," said Mallam Adamu. Similar advice is now being given to combat the AIDS epidemic, the modern equivalent of syphilis. I doubt if my advice was heeded, though, as when asked how he had spent one holiday weekend, he replied "I spent it dancing with the harlots."

When I first arrived, I asked for intravenous fluids for a severely dehydrated man with gastro-enteritis, to be told that they were unknown. I found one giving set and two bottles of saline in a store cupboard and used them successfully. As dehydration was a common cause of death, I re-used the set numerous times and had to make up my own saline solution. We had large salt tablets of known strength in the dispensary and boiled them up with approximately the correct amount of filtered water with excellent results. The reaction to the inevitable impurities was of little consequence as the patients survived. I later read of intravenous coconut milk being used in India, another example of using local materials successfully in desperate circumstances.

Soon after arriving, I prepared a submission for increased funding, and doubled the drugs and dressings budget, so we could phase out NAB and use penicillin. We spent a lot of money on dressings, much of it for tropical leg ulcers, which a third of the population had had at some time. With anaemia from malaria, hookworm and other parasites, a marginal protein diet, and lack of many vitamins, a graze on the ankle quickly became infected and ulcerated. The nursing staff operated an ulcer-grafting system. The head nurse gave a quick anaesthetic with open ether-chloroform mixture, and the theatre nurse curetted or cut out the chronic ulcer, and took a skin graft from the thigh with a Humby knife, a surgical cheese slicer. The graft was put in sterile saline and kept in the fridge for a week, whilst the ulcer bed was cleaned up and kept untouched, with a simple dressing of penicillin powder and Vaseline gauze. After one week, the graft was applied to a surprisingly clean ulcer bed, and rebandaged for a further week. The nurses became very skilful and the majority of the patients were cured, until their next injury, just as the gonorrhoea cases were cured until their next infection.

There were times when I felt I was just scratching the surface, and the real problem lay in educating the public. However, I was encouraged by a visiting doctor who told me about the successful Yaws eradication program in the steamy Niger River delta. Yaws is a spirochaetal disease not unlike syphilis but not sexually transmitted. The infection was widespread and treatment with one injection was given to everyone in the region. The doctor and his assistants sat in one canoe, and the villagers would glide past in theirs, sitting on the edge, perfect targets for injections into their hips, an effective medical mass production process, known as "bum-punching".

At the end of the dry season, with the dust storms came two major epidemic diseases, smallpox and meningitis. I arrived shortly before a large scale meningitis outbreak, without appreciating its potential havoc, having seen only one case in England. Ten or so villagers in each village were infected, and were being nursed by the dispensary attendants in separate straw huts, lying in varying levels of coma, heads pulled back with the characteristic neck stiffness.

The only medication we had was sulphadiazine in tablet form, but difficult to administer as most patients were unconscious and unable to swallow. So we mobilised as many paramedical staff and village heads as were capable of using syringes, and boiled up fifty tablets each in clean used beer bottles fitted with rubber caps and taught them to give injections into the upper buttock, half way between the sciatic and femoral nerves. Naturally, tablets are not designed for injection, but we had no choice if we were to save any of those desperately ill patients. Our teams set out with their primitive therapy, and saved a number of early cases, as sulphadiazine was a very effective drug. The sterile abscess at the injection site was a small and treatable price to pay for life.

Early in the wet season, smallpox outbreaks were reported from outlying villages and triggered a flurry of public health activity which I could not at first understand. I had not appreciated its high infectivity until I visited villages where many lay dying, their bodies covered with purulent sores. Again, teams were sent out to vaccinate as many uninfected people as possible.

Even in the early stages there was time between contact and the fully developed disease when vaccination could modify its severity, but it was useless after the rash appeared. We had only general supportive measures, plenty of fluid to balance the fever and sweats, and swabbed down the open sores with a sulphadiazine paste to diminish secondary infections. One quarter of the patients died in this outbreak.

A leprosy village had been built half a mile from the hospital. I visited it monthly, a most depressing place with about a hundred lepers and their families existing in an atmosphere of fatalism and quiet despair. They showed all variations of the disease process, from hands and feet ending in stumps without digits, to the lion face of a young man in the acute lepromatous stage. The only treatment was to inject around the skin lesions with oil of chaulmoogra, an ancient and virtually useless remedy, long since banished to the therapeutic museum. Four months after I arrived, sulphone, the first effective drug for leprosy, cheap and available in large quantities, was sent out with instructions.

I gave a little speech in my basic Hausa and said that some of them would be going home in six months. They listened with polite scepticism. The next monthly visit marks one of the highlights of my life. The lion-faced man now had normal facial features, and other patients' lumps and bumps were beginning to resolve. Of course, those with lost hands and feet were no better, but the morale of the village had become wonderfully high, so much that I could almost feel it radiating through me. At twenty-four years of age, this was heady stuff, to be honoured for bringing this indisputably effective medicine, albeit by proxy. As word of the successful cures spread, the outpatients increased tenfold. There were many leprosy cases who had kept their skin lesions hidden under their robes, or stayed at home. The morale stayed high, and later, plastic surgeons would become available to retrieve some limb function by tendon transplants, but in 1952, that was well into the future.

There were some dozen outlying dispensaries, which I tried to inspect monthly, visiting a different point of the compass weekly. In the rainy season, some places were cut off by swollen rivers, and I used the ambulance, appropriately called the *"angulu"* or "vulture" which had a better chance of arriving. Once, I was poled across a river in a canoe and then made the last few miles on horse back. My only other experience with horses was as a child, when a massive Clydesdale stallion on which I had been placed for a "nice ride", noticed a mare flicking her tail seductively in a nearby field. He took off through a closed gate and I managed to slide off onto long grass, with a resultant mistrust of horses.

My Nigerian horse was docile, and I rode along regally processing with a retinue of the local Emir's staff to the dispensary in the town. The country people squatted down in deference, or raised their clenched fists, a salute arising from holding reins, unconnected with communism. *"Zaki"*, they called, *"Ranke shedade"*, meaning "Lion" and "May your life be prolonged". Again, this was heady stuff, except that I did not know what difficult and disastrous cases awaited me in the little hut used by the dispensary attendant, and how I was going to treat some abstruse condition with the little experience and minimal medications I had. *"Ex Africa semper aliquot nova"* held a new meaning for me, "Out of Africa always something new".

At one dispensary, there might be two or three large abscesses for incision, many enlarged malarial spleens, numerous coughs, among which were one or two cases of tuberculosis. This was another plague, as the Africans had less resistance than the Europeans, and were difficult to treat, with no antibiotics, nor any chemotherapy. Virtually all one could do was to try to keep them isolated, which was impossible, and to tell them to spit in the fire. The only cases I ever managed to treat effectively were either rich merchants who could afford it, or officials and policemen who could be followed up.

At Shira, a small town set prettily amongst huge granite boulders, the local hyena population had increased so much that the people feared for their childrens' lives. A baiting program was arranged, and I injected lumps of meat with strychnine. Staying overnight in the round mud rest house reserved for visitors, I could hear the animals calling and snuffling around. The next morning, several dead hyenas were dragged in, and a total of forty six kills were reported.

I found the sight of those ugly but magnificent dead animals distressing and never repeated the baiting.

I divided the region into the four points of the compass, each of which had two or three dispensaries, and I set aside one day a week to tour them in the dry season. I took Mallam Adamu with me, with boxes of dressings, medicines, injections, food and overnight sleeping gear. Often, we would hold the clinic on trestle tables under a cool village tree. I was able to do minor surgery such as draining abscesses in the dispensary huts, under local anaesthetic or sometimes pentothal, watched through the window by a dozen pairs of eyes, as very little is private in an African village.

On the way back from one very remote village, miles from any habitation, in tsetse fly and leopard country, the car suddenly veered off the sandy track. The slave arm to the steering had fallen out of its socket and the wheel had turned sideways, fortunately at low speed. There was no chance of any vehicles coming for days. We turned the wheel straight, and lifted the connecting rod back into its socket, and bound it into position with bandages from the medical box. It held together as we drove home, very slowly at first, gradually increasing in speed like a horse sensing its stable is near. This experience increased my respect for the African bush and the necessity for leaving a search and rescue plan with someone.

Jill and I visited one mission station in Bursari, a remote village four hours drive north of Azare, run by an American and his wife. It was very primitive except that they had reasonably up-to-date magazines such as Life and Readers' Digest, and we had been starved of such material in Azare. They also had a superbly well-filled cold store and we had existed on a very basic diet for months, so the meal seemed a feast, with chips and American-style fried chicken.

I settled down to enjoy a few minutes of civilized reading until the missionary said, "It is our custom after a meal, to pray. On your knees, Dr. Jelliffe." I obliged out of politeness but, realising we had a long journey back before the sudden onset of night, driving along unmarked and rarely used bush tracks, we left quickly. I do not know how they were able to cope as they lived in a staunchly Moslem area and had only a handful of "converts", whom I suspect were not genuine, but were being polite.

At the hospital, my confidence with surgical cases increased, mostly because there was no-one else to deal with them. The nearest major hospital was at Kano, two hundred long miles away. Most cases were hernias, hydrocoeles, amputations and a variety of conditions, from tumours of the jaw and mouth to elephantiasis of the scrotum, sometimes down to their knees. The womens' surgery was usually ovarian, large cysts the size of footballs, or Caesarian sections. The anaesthetics were either by spinal injections, local injections, or by a mixture of chloroform and ether, dropped onto an open Schimmelbusch mask by an nurse experienced in gauging how much to give effectively yet safely. The operating theatre was in a separate building with flyproofed open windows, stopping the insects, but not the dust.

An occasional goat would try to wander in, and kept the compound clean by eating organic rubbish, such as old bandages. All water came from a well, and was boiled and filtered before being used for hand washing and sterilisation. I later found out that ordinary well water was often used to cool, and thereby unsterilize this water, but I never had an infected case. There was no electricity, so no theatre light, and no X-rays. In the heat of day, the sweat poured into my operating gloves and I had to lift my hands upwards to allow them to drain. At night, kerosene Tilley lamps were held over the patient with some insects bypassing the netted windows, adding an extra hazard to emergency operations.

The burden of parasites which the North Nigerian had to bear was, and still is enormous. In one small village, I inspected the school children and tested them all for schistosomiasis, a bladder worm which has a complicated life cycle, and is acquired through the skin in stagnant ponds. I collected urine samples from all the children, centrifuged them to isolate the sediment, and added fresh water. After half an hour in the sun, with the aid of a lens, I could see the mobile stage of the parasite swimming about in large numbers. This indicated a hundred per cent infection rate, but I had no medications and to treat every pond in a huge area was impossible. Children will always play in ponds and schistosomiasis will continue to drag down their health by constant blood loss from the bladder.

By the time I had become settled into the hospital routine, Jill, in late pregnancy, was finding the increasing heat hard to bear, lying in a pool of sweat all night under hot mosquito netting. At the end of May, cook Sule had become impossible and was put on a bus to Jos, and we borrowed a cook-steward to tide us over. However, the next day, four weeks before her time, Jill began to get labour pains. While she got ready for the drive to Jos, I collected orders from the other government officers, as a trip to the city meant shopping for the whole station.

This usually included a visit to the local private chemists, Norchem, to pick up fresh supplies of antibiotics which had taken too long to appear from the government stores in Lagos. It was run by an English chemist and his ex-medical student brother who also sold a variety of quaintly named proprietary products. "Pikkino" was for babies' sedation, you could either rub on or drink "Hotto" and the use of "Vomipreg" was self evident.

We set off with the most basic equipment to drive the 200 miles to Jos hospital. By the time we reached Bauchi, she was in established labour, and we drove the last eighty miles with Jill getting more and more anxious. We did not know Jos and first entered the golf club, then an imposing driveway to be greeted by the Resident with his sundowner drink in his hand. In thirty seconds, we had been told the way to the hospital, and arrived thankfully still intact.

I went to the Senior Medical Officer's house to stay for a few days, and around ten o'clock, I was phoned to say that Michael had arrived, needing a forceps lift out, but delivered by a doctor in evening dress dragged from aparty. My feelings were of relief for Jill's safety, and the enormous responsibility of another life to bring up.

Michael was a scrawny premature baby and he and Jill stayed in Jos for six weeks till he had improved. Meanwhile, I had engaged a new cook called David and had done an enormous amount of shopping. On arrival back in Azare, cars converged on our house within three minutes, anxious for news of Jill. We had a little party and toasted the baby with a bottle of champagne, and my diary records Salome, our Persian cat sitting happily on my bed all night, purring in welcome. The new cook David lasted only a short time, as he resented the advent of a woman in charge, and Jill found he ignored instructions in a surly manner. I also think he found the bush setting of Azare lacked any of the more sophisticated facilities to which he, as an Ibo from the South, had been used.

A variety of visitors passed through Azare, mostly government employees. An earnest Nursing Sister came to weigh the infants at the baby clinic a couple of times, and tried to tell the mothers to eat unobtainable citrus fruits to prevent scurvy, not realising that the hot peppers which were used in abundance, have the second highest vitamin C levels in the world. The sleeping sickness medical officer passed through on his way to the endemic areas to our north, where whole villages had been abandoned to that scourge.

The region's ophthalmologist came once to review the local visual problems and demonstrated cases of onchercerciasis, or river blindness, which was to prove useful when I later discovered many cases in Kaduna. He also performed a few cataract extractions, which triggered my interest to perform some myself. The local native practitioners had used "couching", a method of dislocating the opaque hard lens backwards by inserting a needle and flicking it through the supporting capsule, all without any anaesthetic or sterility.

I found an old and rusty set of eye instruments in the operating theatre, polished them up and sharpened the long fine bistourey knife. It should be remembered that the one ophthalmologist was stationed miles away and had a huge number of cases to deal with, so I felt justified in doing this sort of surgery with the youthful confidence born of sudden forced self-reliance. The results were good with no complications in the small number I did. There were a number of old basic thick spectacles in a box in a cupboard in the outpatient department, and I had another Great Moment when my first case, a dignified old gentleman, had his bandages removed, put on the glasses, opened his eyes and said he could see again. It was far more dramatic than curing a hernia.

A young public works department engineer, specialising in well-digging, had arrived from the middle belt of Nigeria to our south, and was staying at Misau, half an hour's drive away. The local dispensary attendant sent a message to say he was sick with a high fever, and at first I thought he had malaria despite being on prophylaxis. He failed to settle with a chloroquine injection and became extremely ill. A rash appeared, corresponding to a tick-borne disease, scrub typhus which I had never seen. Azare was outside the tick area from which he had just arrived, where he had been working deep in the bush. We had only penicillin and sulpha drugs which are useless against the typhus organisms, and I despaired of his life. Then came one of those serendipitous moments in life. In the weekly mail, a small parcel arrived from brother Dick in Ibadan with twelve Aureomycin capsules, a new type of antibiotic, with instructions for their use with newborn Michael in case of some unforeseen infection. I felt that Michael was well and could manage with a total of two capsules split into tiny doses should they be required, so I administered the rest to our well-digger friend. Within six hours, he had a normal temperature and was no longer delirious, making a complete recovery within a week.

We were used to the sound of the ambulance returning from a night's mercy mission, as the driver had a habit of pressing the accelerator pedal rhythmically every five seconds or so, a sound reminiscent of the unsynchronised drone of the German bombers and equally ominous. It would stop outside our house, and Mallam Adamu would whisper at our bedroom window, "Excuse me, Doctor," until I came out. This also gave time for the unofficial fare-paying passengers who had strained the springs to their limit over the rough roads, to scatter discretely. This was one of the perquisites to which the ambulance driver felt he was due. Usually the case was serious, as the one and only ambulance was not used for minor illnesses. Vehicle accidents and head injuries sustained in altercations made up the majority.

"He is suffering from restlessness," stated Mallam Adamu, quite correctly, as the patient was convulsing from a severe head injury.

Tetanus is one of the great plagues of rural Africa in the cattle country between the excessively dry sub-Saharan north and the tse-tse fly middle belt. The spores of the causative bacteria lie hidden in animal dung and will not grow in the presence of oxygen. If a leg wound becomes infected with other bacteria which use up the local oxygen, tetanus bacteria can become active and produce their incredibly potent toxin, which passes up the nerve fibres to the spinal cord. The nerves supplying the muscles fire off excessively, and the patient has violent spasms with arched back, sufficient to tear muscles apart internally, leading to death by exhaustion. Most victims had never been immunised and treatment by anti-toxin was usually too late.

Some of the local treatments for wounds compounded the problem. Cow dung was used as a dressing, and also sometimes on newborn infants' navels before the cord had dropped off, adding to the already horrendously high infant mortality rate.

During one morning's outpatient clinic, Mallam Adamu ushered in a quiet, anxious and very hungry Frenchman. Using my schoolboy French, I found he had been travelling across the Sahara by local transport on the way to the Congo, now called Zaire. He came back for breakfast and ate an enormous plate of scrambled eggs on toast, had a bath and slept for several hours. We arranged a more sophisticated method of transport inside a mammywagon cabin instead of on the back, as he left on his adventurous, but foolhardy journey south. But if he made it safely, he would have achieved an experience to last him all his life, and that is really what life's adventure should be about, feeling "the wind in one's hair".

There were a lot of holidays to be celebrated. As well as the standard half Saturday and Sunday of the administration, the predominantly Muslim population had their holy day on Fridays. We also celebrated such British raj occasions as the Queen's Birthday, Christmas, New Year and Easter. The Moslems had the holy month of Ramadan, which varied even more than Easter, and coincided with the very hottest and thirstiest time in 1952 and 1953. Neither eating nor drinking were allowed during the day, so that both patients and staff, except the few Christian southern nurses, became very lethargic and dehydrated. As soon as darkness fell, the town streets lit up with oil lamps, and people wandered about with their friends, eating and drinking until late at night. The most devout refused to swallow their saliva and spat continuously. The really ill patients were allowed to drink, with the proviso that they later had to feed a number of the poor to redress their transgressions.

Towards the end of Ramadan, the first sign of the new crescent moon heralded the general public celebrations of the Moslem faithful and the ending of the daytime fasting. The Emir's district chiefs and their retinues in colourful flowing robes arrived on splendidly arrayed horses to greet the Emir and renew their allegiance in a spectacular manner. The Emir sat in state in front of his courtyard, and the horsemen lined up and charged directly at him, checking at the last possible moment with their reins held upwards in clenched hands, dust clouds billowing about them. The feasting continued into the night, with dancing to the drums which the African plays so marvelously. Once more, I had sleepy nursing staff in the morning.

Ramadan was the annual meeting time for the mostly nomadic Fulani, who drove their cattle back and forth across the country as the seasons changed. The young men came to prove their manhood in a violent way before they were allowed to marry. A Fulani carries an inch thick staff of his own height to help herd his cattle and as protection. Groups gathered around a young man bare to the waist, with feathers and coloured bracelets adorning him. He held aloft a small mirror to look at himself, whilst his friend would make pretended swings at his torso with the staff. He was not allowed to flinch even when he was finally hit as hard as possible, two or three times. They often chewed datura seeds, which had a mitigating effect on the pain, an equivalent to a "trip" on cannabis. The scars were proof of his manhood, if he did not succumb to his injuries, such as a ruptured spleen, which was usually enlarged anyway from malaria. It was the Fulani equivalent of the manly scars sustained in a football game in Western cultures.

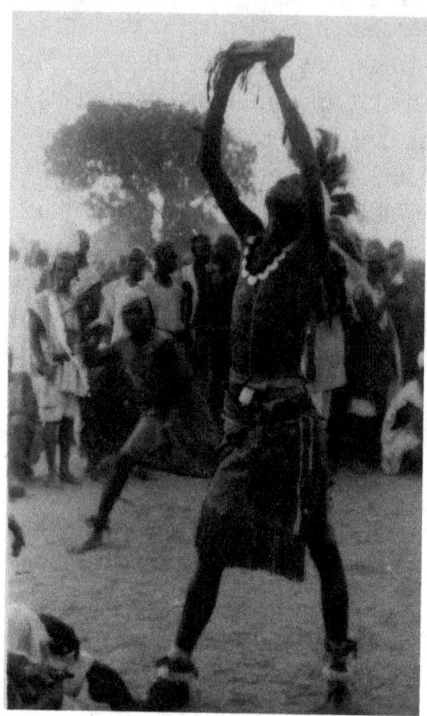

Fulani man proves his manhood with a ceremonial beating, 1953

The pre-marriage dances were equally exciting but less traumatic to the participants. The young men in their finest regalia lined up opposite a row of attractive young ladies who were giggling and simpering hopefully, their hair tied up in neat well oiled parcels. The men wore large loosely fitting thongs on their feet and when the dance began, they drummed them on the ground in a stirring syncopated rhythm. This had a similar effect on the young women as a row of tap-dancing chorus girls has on young male theatre goers, with a mutual sparkling of eyes leading to longer lasting unions.

Hunters brought in a baby gazelle, which had been abandoned by its mother as she evaded capture. They knew that Europeans, and especially the women, loved baby animals and sold it to us. Gazelles are difficult to bring up, usually dying of constipation, so we added a lot of sugar to its milk knowing this gives human babies diarrhoea, and had no problems. We created much local interest during our evening strolls, with Michael in the pram followed by our two grey Persian cats and the gazelle running wildly back and forth, occasionally leaping gracefully over a bush, before coming to heel with its little tail flicking over its white trousers. The women returning from market with enormous bundles of produce on their heads watched with amusement but still managed graceful, perfectly balanced curtsies. We reared it successfully but let it have as much freedom as possible. When the herds came near in the rainy season, it became increasingly restive and finally joined them.

As our second hot season approached, we decided that Jill should go back to England early, as she had become pregnant and needed building up after nearly eighteen months on a basic diet. We were due for local leave and decided to spend it near Jos. Michael had his yellow fever injection there and had to wait ten days before being allowed into England. We stayed at the Veterinary Department's research station at Vom, a few miles out of Jos, in clean, basic accommodation.

We explored the extraordinary lunar scenery of the Jos plateau, a tropical Wuthering Heights, with huge outcrops of boulders on a forbidding landscape under an enormous sky. The final leg to Kano to catch the plane was on the dry season road, with potholes hidden under sand. One depression was so deep and sudden that all the stores we had bought for Azare's residents cascaded forwards onto Michael in his carry-cot. We uncovered him unharmed from under a pile of vegetables and tins of meat, and slowed our pace.

We had to cross several dried up sandy river beds into which we charged as fast as was safe, hoping to avoid becoming bogged. In Africa, however deserted a place seems, there are always helpful local people happy to push vehicles out of such situations.

I saw Jill and Michael off at Kano Airport on the night flight to Tripoli and London in a BOAC airliner powered by four Rolls-Royce Merlin piston engines, which gave me a great sense of confidence. In the days before jet travel above the weather, the night flight avoided the extreme turbulence from the Sahara desert. By an extraordinary coincidence, she had a seat on the aircraft next to a couple whose parents had sold their house in Wimbledon to my father, where Jill would be staying.

I returned to an Azare without females on the Government station. We had a different district officer and two assistant DOs. Hector was a tough bachelor who prided himself both on his iron constitution and his invulnerable digestive tract. Our little band met every weekend to drink gin and bitters, and play the gramophone whilst we solved the insoluble problems of empireminding and discussed the finer features of the district officer's wife at the next station, Potiskum, known to Hector as the "Potiskum Potato".

The coronation of Queen Elizabeth II was celebrated throughout the far corners of the then British Empire, and Azare was one of the farthest. The district officer and the public works department set up batteries of fireworks on frames on an area of open ground outside the town walls, anxiously watching the weather as it was the beginning of the rainy season. During the day, weatherbeaten hunters held archery contests in a surprisingly accurate fashion, considering the arrows had no guiding tail feathers. Wrestling was popular, the contestants vying to snatch a piece of coloured cloth from their opponents' belts, with no serious injuries nor loss of temper involved. The government departments formed teams for the only foreign sport, the tug-of-war. As night fell, speeches were made wishing the new Queen well, and fireworks lit up the sub-Saharan sky to cries of "Yahweh" and "Mardalla." Our little group of expatriates retired to the DO's house to continue drinking Her Majesty's health, and listening to the drumming from the town.

After eighteen months, it was time for my three months leave. I packed up all my gear and drove to Kano to store the car and take the plane to England. I had arranged to stay in Malta for a week to revive childhood memories. Guided by vaguely remembered place names which were spelt totally differently on the map, I wandered the streets of Valetta, saw the flat I lived in twenty years before at the age of five, and caught the ferry to the little island of Gozo. I bought a very superior Italian snorkel face mask and spent hours lying face down over the rocky inlets, retiring with a sunburnt back and a mild case of sea-sickness from the constant rocking motion. I visited Hagiar Qim and its ruins, but never found my Teddy bear.

On arriving in London, I spent the night at my father's house before taking the train to Somerset where Jill and

Michael were living with her parents in their fifteenth century thatched cottage. After the drama and two hundred mile dash at Michael's birth, Jill swore she would stay within walking distance of an English maternity hospital, and we did exactly that. Tony and Joan were looking after a friend's house and we used their London flat, a hundred yards from the Middlesex Hospital for the next three weeks, during which time Peter was born with no problems. I then did a two week locum for the ophthalmic resident doctor hoping to be able to use any expertise so gained during my next Nigerian tour of duty. It was most interesting but of no use as Kano, where I was next appointed, had the only large eye facility with two specialists in Northern Nigeria.

As Jill had never seen Malta, we spent the last two weeks of leave there, en route back to Nigeria. Fog delayed our flight out of London and we arrived late at night, Jill tired and thirsty with two small babies and irregular meals. The water was very saline and we relied on bottles of soft drinks after a disastrous underestimation of the strength of the local wine which saw Jill lose her bearings in the hotel corridors. We hired a car and revisited the neolithic temple and beaches, and the old Knights Templars' fortifications around Valetta. We later had a short flight to Tripoli where the airline put us up in a very plush marble hotel till the midnight flight across the Sahara to Kano. Jill disposed of a paper nappy down the toilet, which had very narrow pipes resulting in a minor flood. Whilst we were waiting at the airport, there was a power blackout, leaving Jill in total darkness feeding Peter in the ladies' room. We were glad to lift off again en route for Kano.

Chapter 7: KANO AND KADUNA

The four Rolls-Royce engines droned on encouragingly over the Sahara desert. The endless sand dunes and stoney ridges gave way to patches of green and occasional clusters of thatched round houses. In the early morning light, the note changed and the rush of air quietened as we began our slow descent into Kano city. The more experienced travellers strolled to the wash rooms to freshen their faces and empty their bladders as customs delays frequently occurred. As the plane's doors opened, a blast of ovenhot air hit us. "We're back," said Jill, her face shining more with perspiration than anticipation. "At least we're in a larger centre."

Kano is the biggest sub-Saharan city. Timbuktu used to be its equal but its population had shrunk to 15,000, whilst Kano had 120,000 people in 1953 when we arrived. It is a thousand year old city, its twelve mile long walls enclosing enough arable land to supply it with food during a long siege. Outside the city lies another town, the Sabon Gari or New Town, in which the large number of Southern Nigerians lived. The higher educational facilities were mostly in the south and hence many of the minor administrative jobs were then held by southerners, Ibos and Yorubas.

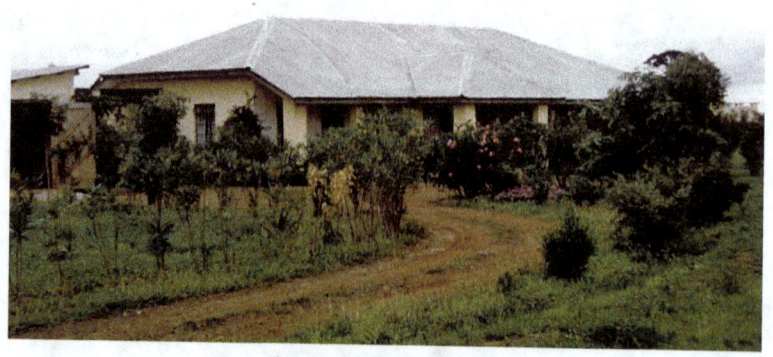

Our house in Kano, 1954

The houses were built in the traditional manner with walls of a mud-straw mixture which just lasted through the wet season and were renewed during the dry. The rich had cement rendering applied to prevent excessive wash-away. The city itself had many ponds between the roads, the source of building mud and mosquitoes. All had flat roofs with little dog-ears at each corner and were cool and comfortable inside. The main buildings were the mosque and the hospital, built of concrete block to public works specifications, and the Emir's palace in traditional mud brick with a large enclosed courtyard, opposite the administration complex.

The hospital had 300 beds and drained a population of over a million people. It had long concrete block units, medical, surgical, female and maternity, with two operating theatres. There was a basic X-ray unit, a pathology laboratory and a pharmacy. Outpatients were seen in two small rooms with queues stretching back along the verandah. The nurses identified the acutely sick who were seen as quickly as possible. Rapid examination was necessary to service the large numbers and most diagnoses were on clinical grounds. X-rays were mostly chests and fractures. Pathology, as would be expected in the tropics, concentrated on blood counts and parasitology.

As in Azare, I started early and processed as many outpatients as possible, before starting an operating session which sometimes lasted well into the afternoon. Injuries made up a large proportion of the acute work, either horrific lorry accidents with outside passengers being flung off at high speed, or the results of violent arguments with sharp or heavy blunt instruments.

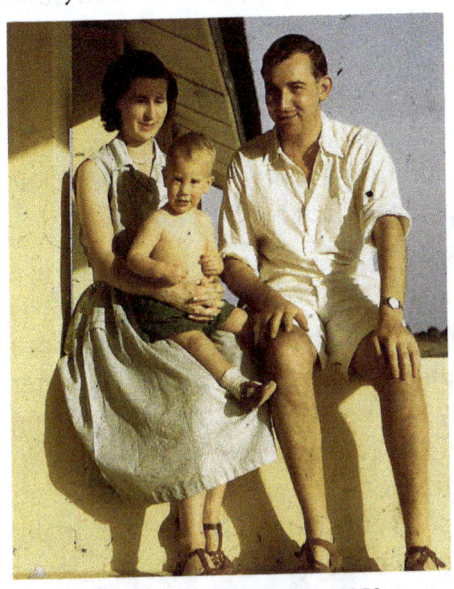

Jill, Michael & Robin, Kano 1953

Scrotal elephantiasis and hernias down to the knees were common, strangulated hernias being the second most common emergencies. Appendicitis and peptic ulcers were rare, possibly due to the mainly vegetarian diet, and the relaxed attitude to life.

In the synthetic capital, Kaduna, my next station, whose civil administrators had a more western style diet, appendicitis was more common. There were a few oddities, such as a parasite which lived in snake lungs in Southern Nigeria, and whose eggs were coughed up into river water. Drinking the water or eating the snake resulted in the larval form hatching and creeping around the abdomen. Being in the wrong host, it eventually died but caused ulcer-like symptoms and showed up as small calcified crescents on X-ray.

I performed at least two leg amputations every month for perforating ulcers or malignant change in chronic ulcers.

These were followed up by a unit which made simple peg legs. Frequently, problems which had to have immediate decisions made work unpredictable.

A man walked in with the aid of a stick with a discharging sinus in his lower leg, which appeared to be due to osteomyelitis, an infection of the bone. I had seen many of these and usually managed to lift out a sliver of dead bone to allow the wound to heal by slow granulation. As I incised over the infected area, the whole of the last four inches of the tibial bone came away in one dead pipe-like piece, leaving an impossible gap between the unaffected ends. There was no other solution but to amputate the foot which had been left dangling precariously supported only by the thin fibula.

There was no blood transfusion service and I had to use relatives if available. I gave a baby whose blood was 30% normal a small transfusion from the donor mother whose blood was 70%, there being no-one else available. Another man came in with a badly crushed leg which had spreading gangrene up to his knee. He refused amputation and two days later, gangrene, (death of tissue within the living) had reached mid-thigh with a severe toxic anaemia. He finally agreed and I asked the male nursing staff for blood donor volunteers. Most of them hid, or stated "I have fever" or "I am weak today" and I do not blame them as this was an intrusion into their personal lives. One male nurse finally agreed and anxiously gave a pint of blood, luckily the same group.

The patient survived and the local newspaper told the story, "whereupon, Mallam Musa volunteered to give blood." I did not grudge him his moment of heroism as he had been the only one with sufficient courage to do something which was quite foreign to him. I brought up the possibility of starting a transfusion service with one of the Emir's religious advisers, but he declined to sanction it, despite the transfusion service present in Mecca. Perhaps he was right, as there were no other tests for the large number of potentially dangerous diseases which are blood transmissible. AIDS was unknown, yet one of its common final events, Kaposi's sarcoma, a blood vessel cancer, was frequently seen.

The Government housing estates were outside the city walls, and we lived in a two bedroomed bungalow in an area which became a lake in the rainy season. In the dry season, we had the usual struggle to keep the small garden alive with bath water.

Drumming from a village half a mile away kept us awake till late, and I was warned that it was a thieves' den. As in most houses, we had expanded metal, a type of thick steel mesh, on the windows, with a small opening for the latch. Experienced thieves put their arms or a stick through this and lifted articles of clothing. They often put razor blades in the sticks to discourage retrieval of stolen goods. One story was told of a tough African woman who grabbed an arm and chopped it off with a sword she kept beside her bed.

I had two deterrents. I paraded conspicuously with my .22 rifle, and I piled empty baby food tins on the inside door handles so that the slightest attempt at entry would make a clatter and wake us up. I slept with my rifle beside the bed and was aware of any odd noises, except the baby's. Jill had the opposite noise sensitivity. One night, I heard suspicious sounds from our neighbour's house, fifty yards away. I tiptoed out and approached a figure prowling around his garage. He saw me about twenty yards away and I fired several shots over his head as he ran like a startled antelope, clearly visible in the full moonlight. My neighbour had also heard him and was creeping about. He was even more startled by the shots, but we were never bothered again.

For the first time in my life I had private patients amongst the Syrian and Indian merchants and wealthy Hausa trading families, visiting their homes with my bag of injections and other tools of trade. The traditional Levantine hospitality meant an invitation to drink a sizable glass of whiskey, which I politely declined but accepted the offer of Coca-Cola. This was almost as dangerous as I was presented with two king-sized bottles. One day, I visited three such families, and, awash with fluid, I vomited blood, since when I have had a great respect for this world-wide beverage, whose exact formula is a trade secret.

I also held clinics for hundreds of Mecca pilgrims, who had to have international certificates for cholera, smallpox and yellow fever. They were sent by lorry hundreds of miles across the sub-Sahara, having saved up for years to make this sacred journey. Some perished on the way there or back and the poorest ones had stories of being charged to sit in the shadow of trees outside Mecca houses. The more wealthy took chartered aircraft, old Bristol Freighters, which could not climb above the turbulence arising from the desert. Air crew told of passengers squatting in the aisle to make a cooking fire, or to pass urine, with airsickness on every trip.

Our hospital lost its chief nurse in Mecca, either from heat stroke or a heart attack whilst he was circling the Ka'aba, the sacred black stone, with thousands of other pilgrims in extremely high temperatures. He had been the chief anaesthetist, an expert in the use of ether-chloroform mixture poured onto an open mask. On a previous pilgrimage, he had saved a life by draining a gangrenous strangulated hernia with a knife, using a small quantity of chloroform, allowing time for arrival at a hospital.

His place was taken by Mallam Habu Challowa, a small, dignified and experienced nurse who looked after me in his quiet way, gently suggesting modified methods of treatment when he saw me getting out of my depth.

One of my other duties was to conduct postmortems, mainly for coroners' cases. Usually, these were straightforward, but one case I declined, was a beggar found dead in the street. He was probably a schizophrenic, for which there was no available treatment, and was wearing strange bangles and head gear. I thought at first that he had been covered in dirt, until I realised it was a moving mass of lice.

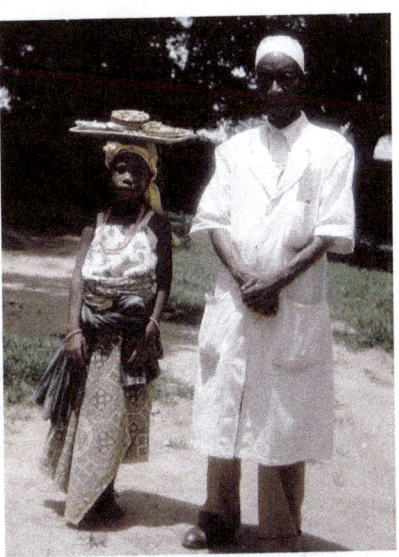

Head nurse Mallam Habu, with daughter, Kano, 1954

Twice I was asked to do exhumations when there had been accidental road deaths. The first was of a man who had been buried beside the road by his fellow villagers, as was the Moslem custom. However it was not the custom to dig up the dead, and I had an escort of armed police, surrounded by a very angry crowd. I did the quickest and most useless examination, gagging with the pungent smell of the badly decomposed body as it would have required a London forensic specialist to interpret the semi-liquid remains. The other man had been buried with many others in an unmarked graveyard. A distant relative made a questionable identification of the spot. I knew the victim had a fractured femur, and as my exhumed body did not, we gave up.

The other doctors in Kano were not interested in surgery and were happy to leave me the majority of such cases and I became interested in the plight of women with vesico-vaginal fistulae. This is a condition where there is constant leakage of urine from the vagina through a false passage. There were two main causes. Girls at puberty were married whilst their pelvic outlets were still immature, and often had four or more days in obstructed labour. The baby was always dead and the constant pressure of its head had necrosed a large hole in the front vaginal wall into the bladder. The older women had a different cause, namely the internal cutting by a female unqualified practitioner, for unexplained loss of the periods, if pregnancy had been ruled out. This left a neat, easily reparable hole into the bladder. The other ones were impossible to repair, being huge and scarred, and I resorted to transplanting the ureters, the tubes from the kidneys, directly into the lower bowel, which gave them some control. There must be thousands of these unfortunates in Africa, living short hellish lives, despite the recent improvement in surgical repair procedures.

A much needed orthopaedic surgeon arrived and soon began a romance with a young sister, eventually going on leave to marry her. He took his honeymoon in the French capital, and I had great pleasure in sending him a telegram of congratulations: "Don't get plastered in Paris". I also had charge of the nursing home, which acted as the hospital for the government officials and their families and any private patients. One of my early patients there was Jill. Our old friend Sylvia, from Azare days, had contracted infectious hepatitis-A the day before leaving for England, and we looked after her children. Thirty days later, Jill had a fever and became jaundiced, and our neighbour looked after our children. Thirty days later, she too became jaundiced as did the next carer. We had no prophylactic gamma globulin in 1954.

Peter became a victim of the Tumbu fly. He had slept in nappies onto which some fly eggs had been laid whilst drying on the clothesline. These hatched out and a few tiny larvae entered the skin of his bottom where they grew into miniature grubs, which looked like blind boils. Careful examination of the top of the reddened areas revealed the breathing end, and a wipe with vaseline caused the larva to retract to clean itself. The grubs were squeezed out with a lot of force but the area never became infected. From then on, Jill ironed all nappies with a very hot iron.

Kano is a city full of character and tradition. When Saharan caravans arrived at the old city gates, they were greeted by lookouts on camels, blowing monotonously on eight foot long trumpets. This custom was continued at the airport for incoming aircraft, and made excellent travel photographs for tourists.

The old Emir had died recently, and through one of his relatives, a nurse, I was able to become an official photographer at the magnificent inauguration ceremonies, when the district heads came to greet their leader. They arrived in brightly coloured robes and turbans, seated on splendid Arab horses, often wearing chain mail, heirlooms which may have been Crusader in origin, with traces of crosses still visible on their shields. For such an important

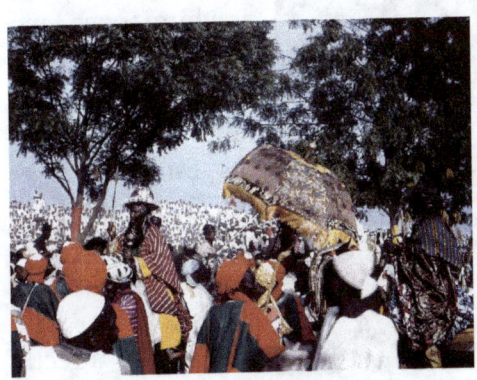

Procession of Emir of Kano, 1953

occasion, Emirs from as far away as Zinder, of Beau Geste fame in French territory to the north, converged on the city's large square. Dust, colour and the braying of trumpets made an unforgettable scene.

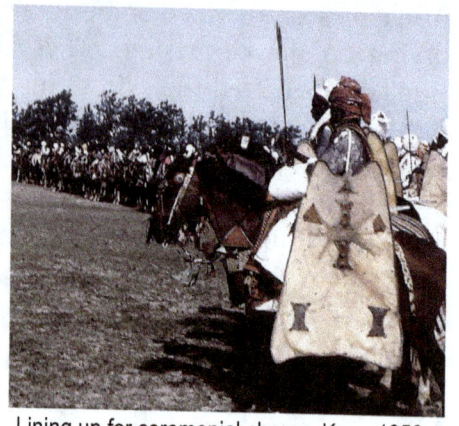

Lining up for ceremonial charge, Kano 1953

The Emir himself, in yellow robes with a red and white striped cloak, rode between his body guards who were clad in distinctive red and green and twirled a large embroidered sunshade above his head. He was followed by a retinue of court dignitaries, a spare horse and the court jester in an outlandish shaggy garb whose function was to ridicule everyone, including the Emir, without fear of reprisals. White-robed subjects covered the city walls as the procession approached a covered dais. The visiting Emirs and district heads waited with the British Governor, who was wearing his full ceremonial dress, magnificent, but rather portly in white, with a white topee and a row of medals. Each district head knelt in front of the Emir and gave his allegiance, then the horsemen lined up two hundred yards away and charged directly at him, stopping

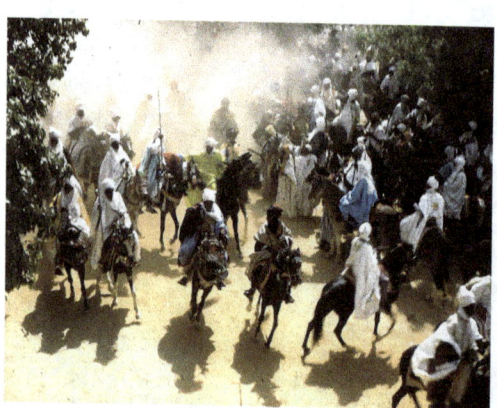

Charge of Emir's Chiefs, Kano 1953

Sparrow in the Hall

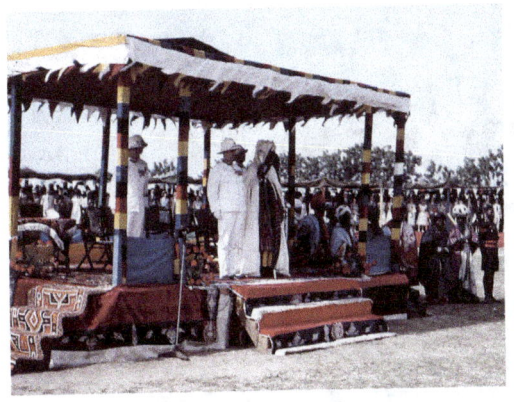

Emir of Kano with British Governor

and rearing up at the last moment, holding a spear or sword aloft as a salutation, a fitting end to a day full of pomp and ceremony. Shortly after this, I was transferred to the administrative capital, Kaduna.

Kaduna, meaning crocodiles, long since converted to hand bags, sits beside the river of the same name. It was built by Lord Lugard as an artificial capital for Northern Nigeria, in territory unconnected with any major tribal group. All the main houses were of European design, usually concrete block, and we were given one of the original houses with upstairs bedrooms. It was a short stroll past huge frangipani (*plumeria*) trees and a well established garden of tropical shrubs to the Government nursing home, where I was in charge. Here, I held a daily outpatients clinic, and looked after the inpatients, both surgical and medical.

I had other duties at the General Hospital, mostly surgical, and helped out with an outpatient clinic, sim-ilar to Kano.

I was also the prison doctor. Kaduna prison was very different to the easygoing, almost holiday camp atmosphere at Azare. The long-stay serious offenders were incarcerated in a large compound behind high thick walls and a heavily barred entrance. Most had long sentences, and there was no evidence of letting the town ladies in, nor were they allowed out as working parties.

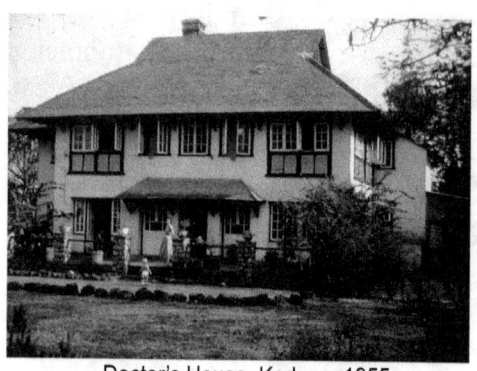
Doctor's House, Kaduna, 1955

It was also the execution prison for capital offences, and I had to be the medical witness. There were two gallows rooms side by side, with the condemned cells behind. The side door to the cell opened, two muscular prison warders marched in, secured the prisoner's arms behind his back with a board to keep his back straight, and a black cloth was placed over his head. Trembling with terror, he shuffled with shackled ankles five yards to the platform, a noose was placed around his neck with the knot behind his ear, the executioner pulled a lever, the double doors opened beneath him and he dropped.

The whole process took less than a minute. In a corner of the windowless room, dimly lit by a solitary light bulb, the Moslem priest stood saying prayers, and there was a dreadful close smell of sweat and fear. The victim's fall ended with a snap of his neck, and a loud clink of his manacles, followed by a smell of excrement as his bowels relaxed. The body was left hanging for a few minutes and I checked the absence of heart beats in the room below. It was necessary to do a post-mortem on a concrete slab in the same room, which I did quickly by incising over the back of his neck, confirming the ruptured spinal cord.

It was an unnerving experience, not only to witness the deliberate killing, but also to do a warm autopsy, for bodies normally come from a cold room. Worse was the fact I had been quite friendly with one of them, not realising he was a condemned prisoner. He had been a poliomyelitis victim and had lost much of his muscle strength on one side, including his neck muscles. No account had been taken of this in the calculation of the drop length, so his head had nearly been pulled off.

The prison authorities had arranged for five drops, two at 8 a.m., two at 9 a.m., and one at 10 a.m. I did not eat much breakfast that morning. I witnessed eight executions in my six months in Kaduna, and the only good thing I can say about them is that they are very, very quick. The capital crimes were all murder, and some of them were highwaymen who were farmers in the wet season, and held up donkey trains in the dry. I was told that the British law was used for such cases, but in some Moslem countries, the murdered person's relatives could choose either execution, or to take "blood money" instead or keep the murderer as an unpaid servant for ten years, keeping him fed, housed and not ill-treated, which strikes me as a very civilised alternative.

Poliomyelitis was rife. Many beggars, wasted legs retracted under their shrunken buttocks, used their arms to move about in the dirt. I had one terrible experience at the Government nursing home. A vivacious newly-wed European woman presented with a temperature and a wheezy chest, with apparent signs and symptoms of early influenza. Within twelve hours, she was gasping for breath with polio and had lost most of the muscle power to her chest. The nearest artificial breathing apparatus was sent by some missionaries from Zaria, many miles away. It was a primitive airbag which was fastened around the chest, alternately compressing and releasing. By the time it arrived, the poliomyelitis had spread up to the base of her brain and she never recovered consciousness. The shattered husband told me that he had lost his first wife in exactly the same circumstances three years before.

It is memories of such cases that make me very angry with ill-considered advice from alternative nonmedical sources that immunisation is unnatural. The virus is waiting to pounce out there, brought in by a fly, and respects no social class. Salk and Sabin vaccines have virtually wiped it out from Western society.

Smallpox was the other major preventable viral infection. I gave a lot of spinal anaesthetics for surgery, during which a fine needle was inserted into the spinal canal and local anaesthetic agent injected. A day after doing this on a hernia case in the general hospital, he became feverish and had neck stiffness. At last, I incorrectly thought, I have introduced a meningitis, despite the sterile precautions. The next day a rash appeared in the typical smallpox distribution. I informed the public health department at once, and wondered why there was such a hurricane of activity. I had forgotten just how infectious the disease was. Health inspectors armed

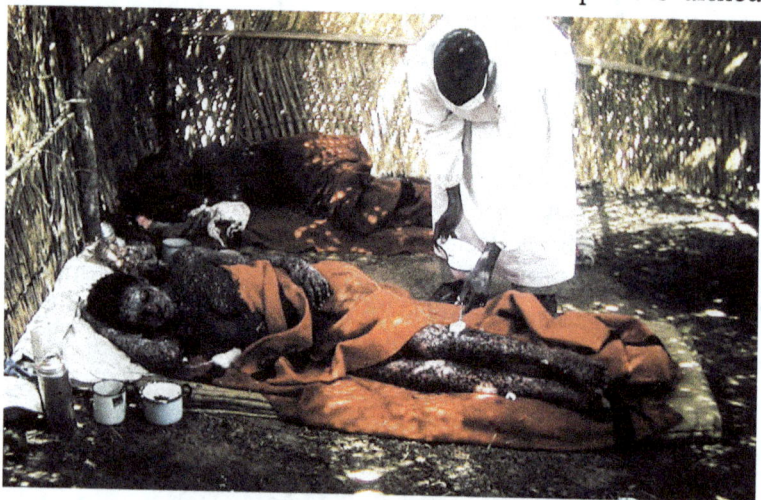

Cleaning smallpox patients, Kaduna, 1955

with vaccine came in through one door to the wards, and some patients, fearful of such procedures, escaped through the back doors.

An epidemic spread through the town and we had to close the main hospital for all but emergency work. I saw outpatients in a house in the middle of Kaduna town, and temporary wards with walls of guinea corn stalks were set up outside town next door to the cemetery. Here we treated and isolated all the cases, and at night one of the nursing staff duties was to prevent the local hyenas snatching bodies, for there was a 25% death rate.

We had a simultaneous chickenpox outbreak, and I had the unique experience of seeing one case of each disease side by side, comparing the rashes. The World Health Organisation later had a major campaign to wipe out smallpox by world wide vaccination, and declared it to be defunct. I hope they are right, as it could spread like a bush fire in a now unvaccinated world if there remains a pocket of live virus in a backwater somewhere.

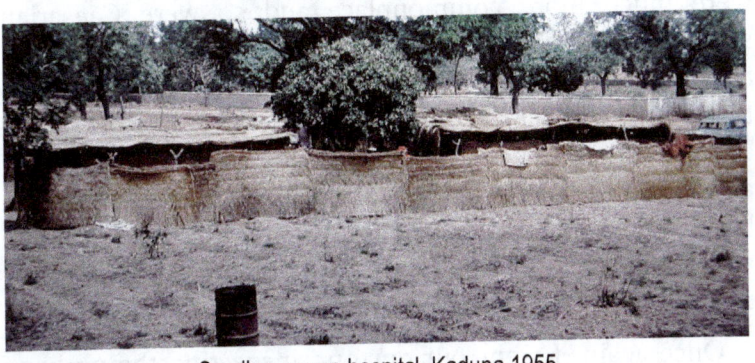

Smallpox camp hospital, Kaduna, 1955

Two young British women secretaries consulted me about allergic reactions and rashes. After work, they spent much time at the swimming pool which had been built on the river bank. I suspected a parasite, *Onchocerca*, which was the commonest cause of blindness in the British Commonwealth. It had been demonstrated to me in Azare by a visiting ophthalmologist. It is carried by the bite of a river fly, *Simulium Damnosum*, and the adults set up perpetual love nests in lumps under the skin, especially on the side of the chest, where they produce millions of microscopic worms, which migrate to the eyes and eventually destroy the retina. The public health department found that 90% of the riverside villagers had positive skin snip tests, and the fly occurred every hundred yards along the bank. Older men were to be seen throwing their fishing nets, totally blind after years of infection. I gave the girls their anti-parasite medication, and as I left for leave, a fly eradication program had commenced.

It was as though Lake Burley Griffin in the centre of Canberra had been infected with an insidious blinding disease, for Kaduna was the Canberra of Nigeria.

I had a series of more western type operations. Appendices were much more commonplace and so were Caesarian sections, one baby being proudly and appropriately named Suleiman el Ksar. One district officer raced back from bush to be with his wife who had had an emergency appendicectomy, and rolled his car. He received a severe blow to the head and became violently confused, walking up the corridors brandishing a loaded revolver, until our tiny Scottish Sister scolded him, "Now, now, we'll have none of that here," and took it away.

Once again, I went out on tour, inspecting the outlying dispensaries. It was at the peak of the hot season and the little villages were surrounded by baked fields which looked as though nothing more could ever grow there again. I went on my own and had to find my way along bush tracks, between and sometimes over granite outcrops, supposedly leopard country.

Once in a very remote area, the car engine stopped on a road over some boulders. The petrol lead had partially blocked with strands of felt which had been used on the petrol tank access cover. I had to open the bonnet every two hundred yards, and manually pump the carburettor full enough for the next two hundred yards. Five miles away, I met the only railway line in northeastern Nigeria, and was able to come back on a flat railway wagon.

The last few weeks before leave, I sold the faithful Standard Vanguard and borrowed a Land Rover from a district officer. Jill was still very low after her attack of hepatitis, and the effects of anti-malarials, so much so that she even had to apologise for not appearing at a Governor's dinner party. We decided to send her back to England early to get the chemicals out of her system in a temperate climate. Shivering, she got out of the plane into the cold March English air and was met by her brother Tony. By evening she was almost paralysed with cold and had to be forcibly marched to her hotel room, and covered with as many extra layers of clothing sister-in-law Jean could find, before being taken to a restaurant. The next day with Michael and Peter she went down to Stogursey in Somerset, to stay with her parents in an old but picturesque thatched cottage. She improved rapidly, her pale tropical cheeks turning rosy pink once more.

I arrived a few weeks later and picked up a little four door Ford Prefect. We spent the rest of our leave moving about the country, visiting Grannie Hebb, staying three weeks in Oxford, then in Wiltshire, and doing a locum in Barnstaple in Devonshire for the elderly GP father of one of my fellow students.

I had reverse culture shock, seeing the relatively minor medical conditions, after Nigeria's sink of serious pathology. I made only one mistake. I was given a tiny Bakelite container with a small electric element in which to boil up the glass syringes in use then. He gave me careful instructions not to let it boil dry, as it was obviously one of his old favourites. The smell of burning Bakelite that evening told me I had failed, and I later had the demeaning experience of a sound dressing down from a bitter old man. I had tried to find a replacement, but it was obviously a treasured museum piece.

Refreshed by our four months leave, we loaded the car on the good ship Apapa and set sail for Lagos with our two little boys to take up the post of Junior Lecturer in Anatomy at Ibadan University for a year, in preparation for the Primary FRCS examination.

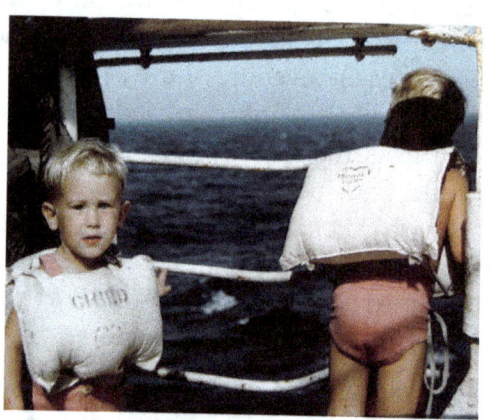

Peter and Michael on the MV Apapa

Chapter 8: IBADAN

In 1955, Ibadan was a huge sprawling city of over half a million, the centre of a rich palm oil and cocoa industry. The new University stood in spacious grounds, modern buildings blending with the surrounding palm trees and lush tropical vegetation.

Overlooking a wide expanse of playing fields, a large well-ventilated multi-storied block housed the library, while nearby, a hall with a theatre catered for the arts. The staff houses were scattered in groups around the edge and we occupied a pleasant two bedroomed bungalow in a quiet backwater.

Brother Dick had left to take up a professorial post in New Orleans, and our neighbours were an interesting cosmopolitan lot, recruited from all over the globe, whilst Nigeria was readying its own academics. In our small road, we had a Jewish physiologist, two New Zealanders, a Swede, a Dutchman and two Nigerians. We waited for several days for our steward, Dogo to appear. He had been waiting near the hospital, and was nonplussed and a little anxious when he found I was working in a highly suspect department, full of dead bodies.

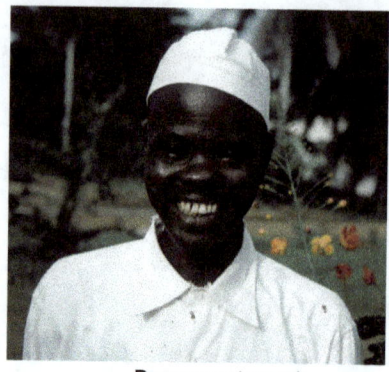
Dogo our steward

The two anatomy, two physiology and single agriculture buildings lay alongside each other on a gentle slope. My professor was an irascible Scotsman who was not on speaking terms with many of his colleagues, including the only other teaching member of the anatomy department, Viv, a quietly spoken senior lecturer from Ceylon. I never found out the story behind this farcical situation, in which I had to play the part of gobetween, forever trying to be neutral. Whenever I talked to one, I could see the other peering suspiciously at me from a doorway.

I heard them talk directly once only. "I'm going on leave tomorrow," said Viv.

"I hope your wife has a good leave," was the instant reply from the professor with his pipe still in his mouth.

The department was affiliated with the University of London and taught to that standard. At the end of the academic year, we were visited by professorial staff from England, who conducted the examinations jointly with ourselves. Allowance was made for the language difficulties, as many anatomical terms were not part of the English taught at school. Having been used to the Scottish, English and Ceylonese accents of our small staff, the students now had to tune in to the different accents of these newcomers, and vice versa. The examiners were generous and relied heavily on our own assessments, whilst keeping up the high standards of the University of London.

Students are the same worldwide, and our Ibadan group had a typical spectrum, from the brilliant to the strugglers. The brightest was a bishop's son, with the advantages of a first class primary and secondary education, which the majority of the strugglers had missed. There were the studious and the sexually athletic, telling similar tales of their prowess to those heard at the Middlesex Hospital Medical School ten years before. My duties were to attend the dissecting rooms, to give an occasional talk about one of the simpler anatomical parts, and to prepare specimens for the museum.

The British Anatomy Act was in force at the time, which meant that any unclaimed body could be used for dissection after forty-eight hours. Many patients with single names came from remote villages and had died without relatives in attendance in the main hospital. So we had a constant supply, which we preserved as quickly as possible with formalin. As we had no refrigeration in the department nor in the hospital morgue, organs such as brains had usually deteriorated beyond specimen status by the time we received these bodies.

I determined to build up a selection of well dissected brains, by calling in at the post-mortem room and collecting fresh specimens personally. These were placed in large earthenware pots of formalin, and taken nonchalantly out by the back entrance to our department for full preservation. I was careful to avoid any contagious cases, but on one occasion, I asked the mortuary attendant for the cause of death. "Fever," he said, and I presumed it was non-contagious malaria. Next day, I found out it was typhoid fever.

In one corner of the preserving room stood a large tank six feet long and three feet high, full of stillborn premature infants, soaking in preservative, a treasure trove for future researchers. In another room, row upon row of skulls sat grinning on shelves, many with their front teeth knocked out, reputedly from the piles of skulls found at the old sacrificial sites. Many of the bodies we received were too decomposed to be of use for dissection purposes, and were skeletonised. The professor had tried many different methods to obtain clean bones. He had two ex- West African Frontier Force sergeants as laboratory assistants, well over six feet tall and fearless. He had tried scraping the bones, and even burying them in ant heaps, finally resorting to removing all the possible meat and putting them into a 44 gallon drum of water with crushed papaws, or papayas. The digestive action removed the last fragments of flesh and the fat was finally cleaned off with spirit, leaving excellent specimens for the students.

The professor had an ulterior motive. He was not on speaking terms with the physiology professor, who seemed to be able to persuade the University authorities to supply his department with any equipment he wanted, including refrigeration, which we so desperately needed. Outside the five buildings, with the anatomy department at the highest part of the slope, lay an open drain. Our professor would wait till a physiology conference was in progress and then remark, "Well, we'd better decant the skeletons today." The drums were upended into the drain and the aromatic fluid would pour past physiology one, physiology two and then agriculture, causing immediate evacuation of their buildings, the agricultural staff being the innocent victims of our internecine wars. Anyone who has ever smelt rotting flesh, even a dead mouse in the wainscoting, knows the dreadful stomachwrenching stench of cadaverine and putrescine.

Anatomy, ten; physiology, nil; game, set and match.

Our department was the one area which was totally safe from thieves. No-one would have dared to go near the house of the dead at night. Another sure burglar-proof ploy was to placean electric light bulb in a skull and leave it at the window. My brother had had a watchdog both as a pet for my sister-in law, who loved "whoofies", and as a burglar deterrent. However, to combat the tendency of animals to disappear, he paid a local witch doctor to put a curse on anyone who might harm it, in a very public ceremony, and managed to keep it for many years.

I kept very gentlemanly hours. The day started with a discussion with either the professor or Viv, the senior lecturer, but never together. I spent much time demonstrating the anatomical structures, keeping one page ahead of the students as they worked their way through the specimens. If they asked me a difficult question, I kept face by saying, " There's a good diagram of that. I'll go and get it for you," enabling me to look up the answer, and accelerating my own learning process. I gave lectures using old Professor Kirk's methods of showing, not just telling, with the extra interest of revealing how apparently dull anatomical facts became relevant in medical practice. Stories of how I was helped by simple anatomical knowledge in difficult situations, whilst on my own in Northern Nigeria, brought home the importance of this basic training.

I had to modify many mnemonics and comparisons to suit the local scene. It was no use describing the prostate as being the size of a chestnut, which they had never seen, but as a kola nut. "Lovely French, etc." became "Lovely Fulani" and "Amiens" became "Abba". I enjoyed the time sitting with them, getting to know their background and telling them mine. It was inter-cultural relations at its best.

We left Ibadan at the end of the academic year, with the job of Casualty Registrar at Nottingham General Hospital to go to. We sold as much as possible, the bishop's son buying all my classical records. I put a "for sale" notice on our little Ford Prefect, and was immediately followed, like a bitch on heat, by dozens of taxis, because it was an economical four-door car, ideal for such work. We spent a nostalgic day in Kano staying with our radiology friend, arriving back in London in mid-summer.

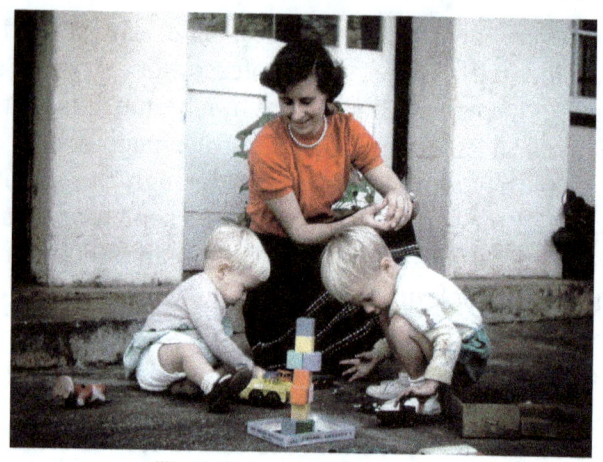

Jill with Peter and Michael, 1954

Chapter 9: NOTTINGHAM AND SHOTLEY BRIDGE

I chose Nottingham for my next post, partly from sentimental reasons, as my mother had been a Nottingham girl, and because the post had been advertised at the right time, and was an approved training post for the surgical fellowship. The board accepted me without interview whilst still in Ibadan as the registrar for the casualty department at the General Hospital, which dealt with over two hundred cases daily. I was the first English doctor there for several years, as these posts were taken up avidly by overseas post-graduate doctors working towards the higher surgical degrees, Indian, Pakistani, West African, Australian and New Zealander. My virtual boss was a retired senior surgeon, who also held the honorary position as Sheriff on Nottingham Council. He had convinced the Sister in charge that I was from Nigeria, and I was somewhat of a surprise when I appeared in the flesh. It was a slight anomaly that a Robin, although not a Hood, should be one of the Sheriff's men. He came in every two weeks, said "Everything all right, Jelliffe?" had a cup of tea and continued his retirement. The system worked very well.

I had two junior doctors working with me on a roster system, with one very long day and night on duty every three days. Our function was to deal with the surgical cases not requiring admission, admit the major problems to the wards, and act as an outpatients clinic for both medical and surgical patients.

Hand injuries formed a large part of the work, as the main industries were coal mining and textile manufacturing. Fingers were crushed between heavy trolleys and the razor sharp rotating blades for cutting layers of cloth lopped off many more. Jill and I went down a coal mine many hundreds of feet below ground level as part of our general education. At one stage, we crawled out sideways from the main gallery in a two feet high seam, with wooden supports holding the roof up, in pools of water and close damp air. We reached the surface with great relief and respect for those miners who spend a third of their lives in such circumstances.

Not uncommonly, I had to deal with evacuation of grease from the palm of a hand, from a high pressure gun which had slipped. The Sister in charge, an overactive birdlike woman, watched me carefully for the first few days, until I tried to remove a fingernail, which I had never had to do in Nigeria. I was not making a very good job of it and Sister said so, so I asked her to show me her technique. From then on we were good friends.

I gave many short gas and oxygen anaesthetics, sufficient to lance abscesses or reduce dislocations. Dislocated shoulders were my favourite and I fancied my prowess at flicking them back into position. Once, I had tried every possible technique to reduce a very muscular man, foot in the armpit, twisting and pulling the arm and turning him on his face. I finally called the petite female Indian orthopaedic resident, who embarrassingly flicked it instantaneously into normal position. We were very careful to identify fingers correctly. My predecessor had been asked by the orthopaedic surgeon to remove the fourth finger and had counted to the little finger. The surgeon had meant fourth digit, the ring finger. From then on, we used the terms index, middle, ring and little and it was suggested market, home, roast beef, none and "wee wee wee" for the toes, from the childrens' poem "This little pig went to market".

Unlike the ward doctors, off duty meant exactly that. I could stop worrying about patients who were not my responsibility once they had been admitted. Jill and I would take the two boys out to a nearby stately home with wide open grounds for picnics.

We played with a balsa and paper glider, to which I attached a tiny rocket motor, with a cylinder of cordite burning slowly inside a metal tube, the hot gases hissing out backwards to give thrust. We tried to find Sherwood Forest as Peter was enthralled by Robin Hood stories, but it had shrunk to a small wood after seven hundred years. However, Nottingham Castle was open to the public and Peter could fantasise there about his heroes.

The Suez crisis, with the attempted British and French reoccupation of the Canal and its subsequent blockage by Egypt, brought on petrol rationing. I bought a bicycle with a 49 cc motor which clipped over the back tyre giving an economical 200 miles per gallon. This left our new Ford Escort van for Jill and the boys, and enough fuel for the 20 mile trip to see Grannie Hebb. It was a miserable time for Jill. We had rented a small house three miles from the centre of town, and suddenly, from being in Ibadan, with many friends and interesting activities, she was in a cultural desert, knowing no-one and without any outside interests, a highly intelligent woman reduced to doing household chores and little else.

Shortly after, my father was admitted to hospital with a lung abscess, due to lung cancer. He settled with antibiotics and radiotherapy, but I knew that his time was very limited. This was the next major time in my life when I felt powerless to prevent death at close range. I found him cheerful as usual, and apparently unaware of the purely palliative nature of the treatment. I know that he was really fooling us into thinking we had been fooled. My mother's radiotherapy treatment, years before, had also been palliative and I do not doubt that he was totally aware of the situation.

During my time at Ibaden, I had been studying for the primary fellowship, consisting of detailed knowledge of anatomy, physiology and pathology. I had one attempt soon after arriving back in England, and failed, and had been sufficiently disillusioned to give up. I was negotiating with West Australia for an assisted passage to Wittenoom, a town wholly reliant on an asbestos mine. I was persuaded to try the primary examination again, and went into the oral examinations totally relaxed, not caring if I passed. The questions were exactly about the parts of the body I had prepared for museum specimens in Ibadan and I answered quickly and correctly with a certain panache. The physiology questions were likewise exactly what I had studied most. At the end of the day, the students lined up and their numbers were called, and to my disbelief, I was told I had passed. This meant that I had to do another year at least, to make up the necessary experience time to take the final surgical examination.

I cancelled the Wittenoom migration plans and looked for a general surgical post, being accepted by Shotley Bridge Hospital in County Durham. That successful examination result probably saved my life, and my family's, as Wittenoom's blue asbestos has been the previously unsuspected cause of deaths from a type of untreatable lung cancer which eventually strangles its victims. The town is at present being destroyed, razed to the ground, a modern day Carthage.

Fifteen miles to the west of Newcastle-on-Tyne, Shotley Bridge Hospital catered for the needs of a large coal mining and steel-working community. It is also one of the coldest places in England, as the warming waters of the Gulf Stream have to pass around Scotland to reach it. To the west of the main town, Consett, the heather and bracken Muggleswick moors lead over the spine of England to the Lake District. Hadrian's Wall and the Kielder Forest, the largest man-made forest in Europe, are within an easy morning's drive.

A solid belt of ugly industrial development to the east provided a source of patients, with our own now defunct steel works belching smoke and tipping red-hot slag onto slopes of man-made mountains. The night sky was lit with a roar straight from Dante's Inferno as the giant Bessemer converter had oxygen pumped through its molten contents. The steel workers had good pay and cosy little houses in 1958. It was a depressed and depressing scene twenty years later when we returned on a nostalgia trip. The steel works were closed and an air of grubby gloom permeated the streets.

Shotley Bridge Hospital had two main general surgical wards, and a large thoracic surgery unit servicing the north of England, which attracted trainee surgeons from many parts of the world. I worked with a Mr. Mackenzie, the Mr. being the title for surgeons, going back to the days when surgeons were not physicians, but glorified carpenters, adept at lightning speed amputations, and blood-letting as a treatment for anything.

Both King Charles II, who apologised for being "a plaguey time a-dying" and Robin Hood were probable victims of the latter practice. Even today, orthopædic surgery is jokingly referred to as "warm carpentry".

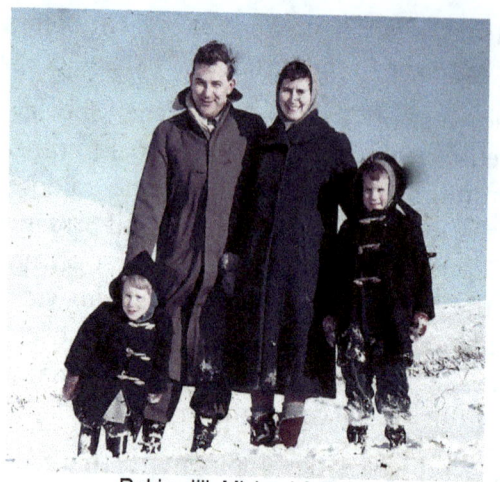

Robin, Jill, Michael & Peter
Muggleswick Moors, 1958

We were lucky to be allocated a small council house half a mile from the hospital, near enough for me to live at home when on emergency call. Each morning, I rode to work on my 49 cc motorised bicycle, which was especially dangerous in winter when the roads were sheets of ice. I spent the day in the operating theatre twice weekly, either assisting Mr. Mackenzie with the major cases—gastric, bowel and thyroid—or performing the lesser operations—hernias, appendices and varicose veins.

Outpatients' clinics, ward rounds and minor operations made up the rest of the time. Once a fortnight, I drove over the moors to a small satellite hospital, to do a list of veins and hernias, operations where there was little likelihood of complications and when Mr. Mackenzie went on holiday, I took the opportunity to do some of the more major cases, gall bladders and acute bowel procedures.

We had to tune in to the local "Geordie" accent, which Michael and Peter rapidly absorbed at the local village school, switching on and off to suit the occasion. One woman from whom I removed a very large fatty flap hanging down from her abdomen, said she had finally come for treatment because a friend had said, "Mary, thou boot sowle's lowse."

She had thought Mary's boot sole was loose and was causing the flapping noise.

I made friends with several of the Indian doctors who were doing their post-graduate training, both surgeons and physicians, registrars at my level and residents on the lower rungs of the career ladder. These doctors, far from their homeland, were tired of the bland and often badly-cooked institution meals, such as porridge and soggy cabbage. To offset this, we held curry Sundays at our little house. They would visit Newcastle for the necessary fresh ingredients on the Saturday, and spent the Sunday morning cooking, midday eating, and the evening recovering.

Role reversal was the rule. I became the junior, peeling the potatoes with Jill washing the dishes and saucepans, many of which we borrowed from the friendly neighbours. Our resident and registrar colleagues became the chefs, introducing us to the excitements of spices and herbs, which, to an Englishman in the 1950s, were still mysterious and deliciously exotic. We soon learnt the techniques and became acceptable curry cooks. We also made a curious curry observation, namely that there was always an abrupt end to the process of eating, when one more mouthful would sink the ship. Each of our Indian friends would stop with a sudden sigh, even with a little left on the plate, and sit back with a happy smile, replete with the taste of his own food. It is no wonder that "curry and rice" has conquered the world's taste buds. Even the Japanese have *"kare-raisu"* high on their food preferences.

My father had been keeping reasonably well, with the effects of radiotherapy holding the lung cancer at bay, but suddenly deteriorated with liver involvement. I went down to see him for the last time in early April 1958, and found him cheerfully accepting his melancholy fate. My brother had been looking after his treatment and eased his passing. I personally could not have been involved in treating my own father and think that Tony had a lot of courage to do so. He died aged 64, on 23rd April, another victim of the cigarette scourge.

He had retired from the Admiralty at 60, and was an executive of a shipping firm. Many years previously, he had worked out how much he would have saved by not smoking, not realising it would include his own life. The effects of smoking and chemicals on the lungs had only recently been recognised. He had asked for no ceremonies or church services, and I respected this with regret. But I still feel I would have liked to have said farewell properly, more than walking away with an aching heart after shaking his thin wasted hand for the last time. I now realise how important some small finalising ceremony is to the grieving process. He missed seeing our third son John, who was born six months later.

There were no prospects for advancement for many years to come with thirty applicants to each consultant surgical post. I looked at hospital positions in the warmer parts of the then British Empire, and was accepted, sight unseen, as medical superintendent by Goondiwindi Hospital, in Queensland, where there was a shortage of doctors. We were sponsored migrants, costing us £10 for each adult, with the three children free, well-known in migrant history as the "ten pound POMs".

The brother of our anaesthetist was in charge of berthing for P&O, and we were given two adjoining first class cabins on the P&O Strathnaver, a totally migrant ship. Farewelled by relatives, including, with great heart-ache, Grannie Hebb, whom we knew we would not see again, we left for Sydney from Tilbury docks on 18 February 1959.

Chapter 10: OUT TO AUSTRALIA

There were 400 Finnish and 600 British migrants on board the Strathnaver, which was on its penultimate voyage before being broken up. We could not understand the formers' speech and had difficulty with many of the latter, who were from Glasgow. I learnt two important Finnish phrases (spelt phonetically) *hoowah minta* for good morning, and *keepis* for cheers. Our upper deck cabins were cool and clean, and the only potentially disastrous situations during that elderly ship's voyage, were a fire in a refrigerator and a flood in the galleys.

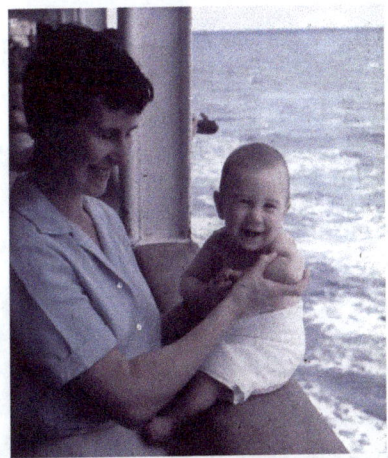

Jill with John on board P&O Strathnaver

Life on board revolved around meal times. Jill would feed five month old John, and would then take the older boys, Michael and Peter, to the dining saloon for their meal. A stewardess would keep an eye on the children while we had ours. We rapidly gained our sea legs and enjoyed the privilege of having an upper deck cabin, rather than the claustrophobic boxes in the lowest decks. After a smooth run across the Mediterranean, the ship anchored off Port Said and started to roll, causing John's cot to fall over and deposit him on the floor. The saloon furniture piled up on one side and the noise of crashing crockery came from the kitchen area. Jill, a dedicated disasterphile, had the boys' escape routes well-planned. We stayed like this until the next day when we joined the southbound convoy through the Suez Canal, with a short stop alongside to lay in provisions.

Our most extroverted Glasgow migrant, the classic loudmouthed thrower of beach balls at the swimming pool, leant over the side shouting insults about Nasser, the Egyptian hero. Fortunately, the local population could understand him even less than we could, or we would have seen him lynched. We awoke with the engine sounds muted, to see palm trees and camels gliding past our porthole a hundred yards away on the canal bank. Halfway through, a squadron of Egyptian MiG jet fighters swept low overhead, proudly reminding us of their victory in regaining control of their rightful territory. In the hazy distance, we made out the the shape of the pyramids.

The air became heavy and humid as we entered the Red Sea. The ship had a following wind so that the cooling breeze of its twenty knots disappeared, and we progressed at a sullen sultry sweaty pace. The passengers no longer strode around the deck, so many circuits per mile, but lounged dispiritedly around the pool and the bars. Even our tactless Scotsman stopped his antisocial attempts at socialising. We watched the flying fish skittering ahead of the bows and had one wondrous moment looking over the side as the ship glided past an enormous segmented fish, a whale shark.

We reached Aden at 2 a.m. in a still oven-like atmosphere. The commercial area was ablaze with lights to welcome twelve hundred potential customers, unaware that most of them were not the big spenders expected from a P&O ship. I went ashore with my shirt soaked in sweat and wandered around the shops on the main street in a dreamlike state and purchased a wideangle lens for my camera. We left Aden at dawn, and once more had a sea breeze to revive us. To mitigate the boredom of the long run to Colombo, the ship's crew arranged as much entertainment as possible, quoits and quizzes, fancy dress parties and bingo, but the days revolved around meal times, not for reasons of hunger, but as markers in the six weeks' voyage.

At dawn one morning, the ship's engines were again muted, and across a faint sea mist, Colombo harbour slowly came into focus, with a golden dome rising above the buildings. We had one day to explore, going to tropical gardens, various temples with the Buddhas reclining in different positions, and finally to the beach at Mount Lavinia and the Galle Face Hotel where our fathers had met during the war. My own father had hated being uprooted at the age of fifty, to leave his family, including his new wife and baby, my half-brother Adrian, and no doubt commiserated with Jill's father, who was his opposite number in the Navy, over a couple of pink gins, perhaps even fantasising over their son and daughter meeting one day.

From Colombo, it was a straight run through to Fremantle, Western Australia, crossing the Equator with the traditional forced merriment and games. Twelve hundred passengers were too many to shave and push off slippery poles, and we relied on our Glasgow extrovert to stand in for all of us. The only other excitements in an increasingly boring voyage, were passing half a mile away from a returning liner which we greeted with blasts on the ship's siren, and skirting the

Cocos Islands, a smudge of coconut palms on a low atoll, on the fringe of a cyclone.

We glided into Fremantle harbour one morning, and went ashore to a totally new environment. It was an intensely hot day, 40 degrees C, and our first exposure to the bright glaring colours of the Australian landscape, so different to the pastel shades of England. We spent one day in Perth, rattling there in an ancient wooden railway carriage, whose sides oscillated sideways, as we passed the dry sandy suburbs with thin-bladed grass and strange new trees. I met my best man, Martin, who had emigrated earlier and settled in Perth. He had arrived with £10 in his pocket, and had found a house in the near suburbs, where there was a shortage of doctors. He put up his plate, found a queue of patients outside the next day and never looked back.

We crossed the Great Australian Bight and arrived in Melbourne on another glorious day, to be met by a cousin of Jill's mother, who apologised for the state of the city, which to us looked like paradise with telephone poles. By this time, Michael had succumbed to measles which had been sweeping the ship in waves. He was being cared for in the ship's hospital situated just above the ship's screw, hot, noisy and claustrophobic, with the bunks and equipment vibrating interminably. Hell for the patients and for Jill who slept next to him. Perhaps it was not really too bad, but we were used to our ex-first-class upper deck accommodation.

Our entry into Sydney Harbour was a magical day. It was early light and the sea was dead calm. We stood at the rails, slowly passing through the Heads, as though we were stationary and the brightly painted houses on the shore line were moving. Our mast passed under the famous bridge with a whisker to spare and we tied up alongside the finger wharf. It reminded me of the old pictures of migrants arriving in

New York, and that we were indeed newly arrived migrants. The organised chaos of customs and baggage collection was efficient, but the health inspector said that Michael would have to be admitted to the Isolation Hospital, being unable to travel with an infectious disease.

Just then, a call came for us over the loudspeakers, and we were welcomed by Graham and Margaret Shirley, friends of Jill's brother when he had been stationed in Sydney, seconded to the Australian Navy years before. They insisted on taking Michael into their home, as they had two daughters of a similar age, who had had measles already, and could not bear to think of him being incarcerated away from home and family on his first day in Australia. He joined us in Goondiwindi two weeks later, flying from Sydney by airline DC3 aircraft. Graham showed me and Peter around the Northern Beaches whilst Margaret took the others to their home in French's Forest. I was dazzled by the bright clear sunny stretches of sand and surf, so different from the grey pebbles of England. It was a great introduction to Australian hospitality.

We rejoined our fellow migrants at the railway station that evening, having already booked a sleeper for the sixteen hour journey north to Brisbane. The train was not designed to give much repose, and we were too excited to stay asleep for long. We stopped at Casino, a small country town, for breakfast, which was laid out on tables on the platform: toast, scrambled eggs with mugs of tea, basic but nutritious. Here, we first learnt the Australian country salute, as the flies descended on our backs, faces and food. After Casino, the train gradually climbed into the hills dividing New South Wales from Queensland and we had the excitement of seeing wild kangaroos, quietly grazing in the early morning sunshine under the gum trees.

At Brisbane station, Jill was left alone with Peter and John, and a newspaper reporter interviewed her as Goondiwindi hospital's new doctor's wife. This was a disaster, as Jill said she anticipated no difficulty there, having been in West Africa previously. This was misconstrued as a socio-economic comparison instead of a climatic one, and caused a few ruffled feathers in Goondiwindi. The photograph coincided with a grimace from Peter, giving the impression of the village idiot. No doubt Goondiwindi society viewed our arrival with apprehension.

We stayed one night at the migrant camp at Kangaroo Point, close to the Storey bridge, a series of long huts with high ceilings and thin eight feet high timber partitions, allowing reasonable comfort, but little auditory privacy. I left Jill, to finish the paperwork associated with registering with the Queensland Medical Board and getting a driving licence and a car. The former was easy and the latter required several trips on foot around the hot streets of Brisbane, trying to convince an uninterested and rather suspicious police department that I was a suitable person to use their roads. I took delivery of a light blue Holden station wagon, of Australian manufacture, and drove it proudly to the migrant hostel.

We left at once, staying the first night at Toowoomba, in the crisp mountain atmosphere. The road from Brisbane to Toowoomba goes west through Cunningham's Gap, a pass in the Great Dividing Range, thence downhill over less and less rolling countryside to the great central plains. We did not turn back, and reached Goondiwindi through a dusty haze in the setting sun the day before Good Friday when all the shops were shut.

Chapter 11: GOONDIWINDI

Goondiwindi lies on the McIntyre river on the Queensland side of the bridge. The name came from an Aboriginal word for the dropping place of birds, where the river-based birds had whitened the tree stumps. It held about three thousand people in 1959, and was the centre of a rich wool-growing industry. It has since changed its main produce to wheat, sorghum and huge areas of cotton, with a cotton gin processing millions of dollars worth each year. At first, the graziers were suspicious of such projects, but finally bowed to the economic pressures and higher returns.

The town itself was typical of the outback, wide streets in a grid pattern, partly bitumen-covered, with the side streets sandy dirt and laterite. Most of the shops were along the half mile main street, food stores, bakery, furniture and electrical, garages for Ford, Holden-GMC, Chrysler and English cars. The Japanese vehicle invasion had not yet begun. The banks and hotels clustered on the main corners, whilst the churches stood discretely in the side streets, the Catholic church claiming the only slight rise.

The medical superintendent's house was opposite the hospital, which lay by the levy bank built along the river to combat the severe floods which occurred every three or four years. We were proudly told the town had recently been sewered and heard tales of raw sewage floating in three feet of floodwater in the past. We had two bedrooms and a sleep-out, a kitchen, dining alcove and a small lounge. The back garden was an arid patch of struggling lawn, full of bindiis with prickles for unwary bare feet.

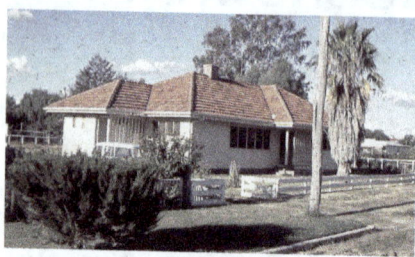

Doctor's house, Goondiwindi, 1959

In the front, a gangly unkempt palm tree harboured a sparrow colony and its droppings. Our neighbour on one side kept horses which later fascinated two year old John who strode fearlessly amongst them. Our other elderly neighbour managed to grow roses successfully.

Arthur, the hospital secretary, a kindly slow-speaking Queenslander, immediately made us welcome. We arrived the day before Good Friday, when all the shops had shut for Easter. Arthur had arranged temporary beds and furniture.

"I've got half a sheep in the hospital fridge for you," he said. We laughed at his supposed joke, having been used to buying four mutton chops in England, but he was right. There it was, with cuts which Jill had never seen before. This was sheep country. During that Easter weekend, sitting around in our bare lounge, one of our new neighbours knocked on the door.

"G'dye, this is God's own country and you've got to have a bit of fish for Easter," he said, weaving unsteadily on his feet, and handed us a large Murray cod, one of the freshwater species found in the inland rivers. We continued to receive such kindnesses from Goondiwindi folk during both our two years there.

The single-storied wooden hospital, since rebuilt, was another typical practical but outdated outback structure, with two main wings, male and female, for mixed surgical and medical cases. There was a balcony at the front, from which the longer stay patients could watch the world go by, or inform the nursing staff when the doctor's infant son, John, had escaped again and was seen heading for the river bank. The maternity ward had been rebuilt quite recently, and was a quiet backwater, joined to the main wards by a covered pathway. The childrens' ward was also set apart, with a small isolation ward. The operating theatre was basically equipped, and could cope with appendices, tonsils, hernias and emergencies. It took five hours to get to Brisbane by road ambulance.

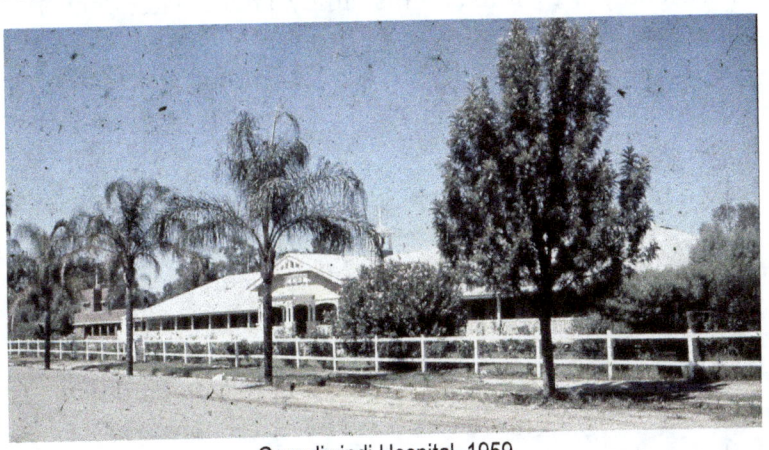

Goondiwindi Hospital, 1959

At the back, the nurses' home, kitchen, laundry and wardsman's house completed the complex. Every institution has its resident character, and we had Jack, the "general useful", to brighten us up. He was a capable eccentric, whose hobby was training polo ponies in an unusual manner. He could be seen riding around, banging drums by the horse's ears, brandishing a tennis racket close to its head and slipping underneath and back again. He assured us this would enable the animal to remain calm in all stressful situations. The nurses occasionally looked after orphaned kangaroo joeys which would hop with them down the outside paths, hoping for a handout. The males became very aggressive as they matured and sometimes attacked the washing on the line, necessitating their expulsion to the bush. By this time, they had lost all fear of humans and probably fell victim to shooters, as their mothers had.

Three other doctors practised private medicine, and I was the "free" hospital doctor, Queensland having had such a system for many years, well before the compulsory Medicare scheme for national health insurance. We became very friendly with Tom and his family, and he later delivered our fourth son Richard, and performed an appendicectomy and tubal ligation on Jill. He left for Sydney soon after we left Goondiwindi, and we have kept up with the family ever since.

The hospital had a series of Matrons, including one with a liking for bottles in her refrigerator whose contents were stronger than milk. The final one was a delightful outspoken English woman who had been Matron of a maternity hospital in Leeds. Between us, we argued fearlessly at the monthly committee meetings against idiotic bureaucratic edicts, as we were not going to be sacked after being brought 12,000 miles, and good Matrons were hard to obtain. She kept two Dachshunds and lost one to baits, which were pieces of food poisoned with strychnine, which some animal hater had left on the lawns. I threatened to leave Goondiwindi as I was afraid toddler John could pick one up, but no more were found so we stayed.

On my first walk down the main street, I was accosted by an outspoken lady in her thirties. "You must be the new doctor," she said. "I can tell by your damn silly Bombay Bloomers," referring to my khaki shorts which I had made in Colombo and which I never wore again. "I want you every evening for the next two months," which turned out to be an unusual way of recruiting new members to the local theatrical group, which I declined.

Characters abounded in Goondiwindi. During the hot summer months, the beer garden of the nearest hotel was entertained by a loud singer of country songs, known as Queensland opera. Her penetrating voice bounced off the hospital opposite and into our bedroom until 11 o'clock, where we were tossing and turning on our sweaty beds. We valued our sleep, myself with numerous night calls at the hospital, and Jill with three little restless children and Rick on the way.

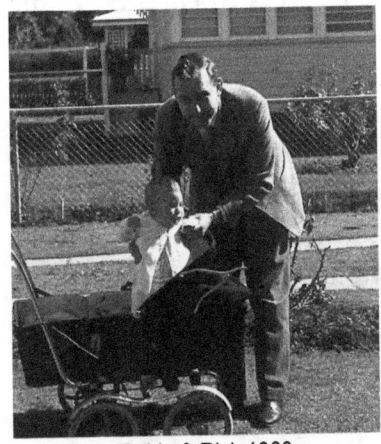
Robin & Rick 1960

Our thoughts were directed vigorously against the source of the noise, and a few weeks later, the hotel burnt down in a spectacular fire. Such was the power of positive thinking.

Subtle language differences soon became apparent. We already knew the story of the Australian school teacher in England telling a student to get some Durex for a torn book, which means sticky tape in Australia and condoms in England. When Jill was invited to her first ladies' meeting, she was asked to "bring a plate", and received a strange look when she asked if she should bring a knife and fork, too.

She turned up with an empty plate, not realising the original request implied cakes or sandwiches.

One evening, Arthur's silhouette appeared through the glass front door, and he said "good night." In England, this is a casual passing remark, so Jill said "good night" and went on with her work, until Arthur added plaintively,

"Aren't you going to ask me in?"

I learnt fast. To be "crook" means to be ill. "Too much condition" means to be overweight, sometimes emphasised with a pat on a protuberant abdomen, for not all Australians fit the lean, athletic surfer's mould, and this expression comes directly from the cattle sales. "Tea" means an evening meal at six o'clock, as distinct from "afternoon tea" at 3 o'clock. To be "gastric" means to have looseness of the opposite end of the gut, short for "gastro-enteritis". One of the classic Australian phrases was graphically illustrated when I was trying to remove some fine stitches from an eye, a very painful procedure. "I hope it's not hurting too much," I enquired. Back came the slow Queensland affirmative drawl, "My word," which said it all.

Each morning, I would cross the road and sit in a hot little office, consulting the "public" patients, as distinct from the "private" ones covered by health insurance who paid to see the other doctors. Many of these had acute or recent conditions, infected hands, chest infections or "gastro". After a few weeks during which the people of Goondiwindi had summed me up and considered me to be, if not brilliant, at least harmless — *primum non nocere*, first do no harm — I attracted a modest clientele of long-term patients, chronic heart conditions, hypertension and even those longest lasting of all cases, skin problems.

With my previous full-time surgical training, I coped with most surgical cases, including Cæsarean sections, gynaecology and tonsils, with Tom giving the anaesthetics. We used spinals, or pentothal with ether, before relaxants such as curare and intubation had become the normal practice.

Country doctors have more than their fair share of emergency work. Car accident victims along remote dirt roads were collected by competent ambulance officers, often with one of the doctors in attendance, and I dealt with numerous fractures. One such case came to see me years later in Coffs Harbour, just to say thanks. He was profoundly deaf and had not noticed the noise of a load of logs, being unloaded from a truck, which rolled onto his lower leg, causing an open fracture. I had immediately soaked the wound in antiseptic and spent two hours delicately bringing the ends together and applying plaster. The other alternative was a long ambulance trip to the city for plating, and I felt the time interval would increase the risk of infection. Most doctors appreciate such thanks, but are slightly embarrassed as to how to reply. To them, it has been another incident for which they have been trained, while to the patient, it has been a huge event in their life story. Nevertheless, a dose of thanks is often a great encouragement to a doctor.

I had a small number of ante-natal cases and deliveries, including a thirteenth child on whose mother I did my first tubal ligation. The father, appropriately enough, was a rabbit catcher. In 1960, Queensland did not allow such procedures except when further pregnancies would have been harmful to the mother. The 1960 AMA Handbook, the little red book of medical ethics, frowned on such practices and the legal aspects were vague, with the husband being in total control of procreation, and his signature was necessary to prevent it. There were and still are civil proceedings possible against doctors who neglect this authorisation as a breach of the marriage contract.

Most partners were only too happy to sign as other methods of contraception were crude at best and unreliable at worst, and the oral contraceptive was just appearing in its original high dose form. A few days after the birth, it is easy to tie the tubes off through an inch long abdominal incision, or nowadays by laparoscopic tubal clips.

I became interested in hypnosis, following the visit of a stage hypnotist, and talks with an accountant friend who practised it. It seemed to have possibilities for the treatment of conditions arising from anxieties. I was well aware that it would in no way take the place of standard ethical medicine but might be a useful adjunct. It turned out to be an easy procedure, especially as subjects trust a doctor to be doing his best to help. I was careful to leave a strong post-hypnotic suggestion that no-one except doctors, dentists or experienced hypnotists could use hypnosis without the subject's full consent. That this was a necessary precaution was demonstrated by a middle-aged woman who came to see me with a broken toe. She had been an excellent subject at the visiting hypnotist's show, and her husband had decided to try his skills. He had left her with her mouth open, unable to speak and she was so angry that she broke her toe as she kicked him.

One young lady who had been an excellent subject during the visit by the stage hypnotist, was admitted to hospital for several weeks to recover from hepatitis, and was happy to try hypnosis for severely sweaty hands, which were causing her much distress. Suggestions to control her own sweating worked for a short time only. I then left the suggestion that she would sweat for five minutes after each meal, thinking that she might have some psychological need to sweat. This worked very well and on discharge, she soon became engaged to her boy friend. I like to think that this might have been due to an increased ability to hold cool dry hands.

A ten year old boy was brought to me as a last resort, before he was to be taken into custody. He had a bad history of violence, cutting up furniture and chasing his mother around the kitchen with an open knife. I put him in a quiet room, in the operating theatre suite, not realising that he had recently had his appendix out there, and was highly suspicious and uncooperative. The more I tried to talk him into relaxing, the more unsettled he became. After half an hour getting nowhere, I said, "I am going to stop now." He immediately went into a deep hypnotic state, as the constant pressure had been removed. Apparently, he stopped threatening his mother, but I do not know if the result was permanent.

It also relieved anxieties caused by a specific past incident which could be relived and deleted from the subconscious. I cured a fear of heights in this way in a friend who had nearly fallen into a deep pit whilst exploring a cave as a Boy Scout. It was useful during labour, but meant getting up at three in the morning to put a mother to sleep. I told one mother, "You will stay asleep unless someone tells you to wake up." Shortly afterwards, the Sister said, "don't wake up," which she promptly did, as the words "wake up" were the trigger. Care has to be used in how instructions are phrased in hypnosis. Generally I found hypnosis to have limited usefulness and phased it out apart from treating bedwetting.

We had several trips to the outlying properties, the Australian word for farms of huge acreages. Tom would stand in for me and we would sometimes drive fifty miles just for a game of tennis and afternoon tea on the little patch of well-watered lawn outside the cool balconies of a rambling homestead. The station cats would respectfully eye off the tame butcher birds and kookaburras which flew up to the tables for pieces of meat. On the drive in, we would see flocks of emus, flicking their ballet dancer tail feathers as they tried to escape us along a boundary fence. Huge flocks of galahs, white corellas and other parrots wheeled over the wheat fields. Kangaroo corpses littered the road's edge, and on the night drive home, we had to slow down, watching for their suicidal leaps into the headlit roadway, where they had been nibbling the small amount of fresh grass on the verges. Others had fallen victim to night shooters, who often aimed at the pinpoints of light reflected from their eyes. This dangerous practice had resulted in the deaths of cattle and sheep and even swagmen.

Feral pigs cause an enormous amount of damage to crops, and are hunted at night with spotlights from the back of "utes", the flat rear half of utility trucks, common on every property. This is a potentially dangerous procedure as the boars are equipped with sharp tusks and the sows defend their young ferociously. More dangerous than the pigs are the shooters with cocked rifles, clinging to the sides of the utes, as they charge across the potholes in the wheat stubble, following a wounded beast. Every year, accidental rifle discharges kill or injure several hunters throughout Queensland.

Feral foxes are also a nuisance, and are shot in a manner of which the English Hunt would not approve. One of my neighbours took me out on such an expedition. He took a four inch square piece of tin plate, snipped a hole in it, and bent it at right angles We drove to a known fox-ridden area, and sat down behind a tree. He blew across the tin whistle, which made the sound of a rabbit in distress, and within a minute, to my surprise, a fox trotted nonchalantly towards us to investigate. Our hunter quickly shot it, and within a couple of minutes, two more appeared, to meet the same fate. He then skinned the heads as there was a bounty on foxes, paid per mask.

Quite early in my Goondiwindi time, I was sent to Mount Macedon Civil Defence School in Victoria, to learn about the atomic bomb threat. I spent a week in a rambling country club with lectures on all aspects of a nuclear war, from ground zero to camp ovens. The only comforting aspect was the fact that generally Queensland was a long way away from anywhere strategic, and fallout patterns from any city explosions would be unlikely to reach Goondiwindi. It felt unreal and academic somehow, but 1960 was the era of nuclear paranoia. I enjoyed the mountains, the first snow flurries on the high ground, and the plane trip over the Southern Alps.

Back in Goondiwindi, I gave a lecture to the local people who, I suspect, felt equally cynical about being able to do anything about such an unlikely event as being "nuked". The main problem would have been accommodation for the refugees from the cities.

The nearest we had to a disaster occurred soon after my arrival. The little tobacco town of Texas, forty miles east of Goondiwindi, was hosting a meeting of farmers, when the stage collapsed, trapping and wounding several. To a new arrival from England, driving along the bush road was another magical experience, with the red dust, gum trees and a kangaroo sitting by the roadside. I went with one of the private doctors to help with the acute needs, giving nitrous oxide sniffs to reduce fractures to transportable condition, and stitching up wounds. I noticed the care with which medical aid was given, but also the careful documentation of the names and addresses by the private practitioners. I realised I was no longer in a free National Health Service area.

All blood transfusions came from a donor panel run by the Red Cross, whilst the important byproducts, plasma, gamma globulins and various anti-sera, were sent out to country areas from the Brisbane blood pool. There was no AIDS nor hepatitis C, whilst the test for hepatitis B went by the name of "Australian Antigen", having been identified first in Aboriginal blood, although, of course, it was found later to be present in many other people. Cross matching from the donor panel was a simple matter of mixing a drop of donor blood with some recipient serum in saline. To involve the country areas and thereby harvest a larger number of donors for the ever increasing demand for blood products, we had a specially accurate refrigerator delivered and organised a recruiting campaign for more local donors. We bled weekly and sent most of the bottles to Brisbane in "eskies"—foam boxes with ice blocks inside.

Television had not yet arrived in Goondiwindi. We had an open air cinema, surrounded by a wall to keep out freeloaders and to allow the resident possums a view of the screen and audience with their goggle eyes. Another resident possum lived above the hospital kitchen. In winter it descended precariously from an upper window every night to be fed with bread and jam by the night nurses wearing thick non-regulation jumpers and stockings, clustered shivering about the fire. The cold dry inland air seemed to pierce every bone in the body whilst in summer, nights were as hot as days and they wore the minimum non-regulation attire.

We were much more social in pre-television days and started hospital auxiliary fund-raising activities. With my supposed expertise in curry-making, I arranged to cook some in two very large saucepans to sell portions to the public at one such function. The graziers' wives chopped and cleaned legs of mutton, and pealed quantities of onions, salty tears no doubt adding flavour to the dish. I left the two containers gently simmering in the care of a friend, who let one of them burn. Burnt curry has a terrible taste and it had to be discarded. The day was saved by adding more lentils and potatoes, and giving Oliver Twist-sized helpings.

At outdoor social occasions, a circle or row of chairs was set up, and the ladies sat together, in their best party dresses, talking babies, clothes, and gossip (or so the men thought). The men coalesced around the bar or beer keg set on a trestle table, talking about sheep, cattle, children and women (or so the ladies thought). My innovative attempts to talk to and even sit beside the opposite sex were regarded as puzzling, revolutionary but acceptable, although I interrupted the free flow of conversationabout babies, clothes and gossip. Jill found that once she satdown on a chair, she was fixed for the next few hours, so shelearnt to choose her neighbours carefully.

Although aviation had always fascinated me, it was not until I came to Goondiwindi in Queensland aged thirty-one, that I was able to handle the controls and learn to fly. An old biplaneTiger Moth would fly for an hour from Inverell with another aviation character aboard, ex-Lancaster pilot Ray McLean. It was equipped with a Gosport speaking tube, which was simply a mouth piece, leading through a tube to two ear pieces in the other flying helmet. We relied on shouting to be heard above the noise of the open cockpit. Ray's diction was blurred and he would say "Mumble, mumble, mumble, HANDING OVER", leaving me with the joystick in hand and no idea what to do. In moments of terror like this, I would stiffen and pull the stick back, resulting in a violent nose-up attitude and roars of laughter from the instructor's seat directly behind me, from which he watched my frightened face in a mirror.

We advanced through the syllabus, straight and level, turns, stalls and spins, landing and taking off, and then changed aircraft to a slightly more modern Chipmunk monoplane, with flaps and brakes, and a voice-operated throat microphone and radio. No sooner had I got used to this, than we changed to the basic Cessna 150 trainer, with which type I later finished my training in Coffs Harbour.

Goondiwindi was a good six hours drive from the coast, and I began to search for a new job. I noticed an advertisement in the local medical journal for an assistant with view to partnership in Coffs Harbour, with a Dr. Rainy Macdonald, so I decided to motor down the coast with a Dutch friend, Pieter Jongebreur, to meet him. Driving south from Brisbane to Coffs Harbour in magnificent weather, we crested around Macauley's Headland to see a gem of a harbour with a jetty sprouting two cranes, and clusters of neat houses. The clean sandy beaches stretched for miles on either side, empty except for an occasional fisherman, whilst rolling banana-clad hills made a perfect back-drop to the scenery. Dr. Mac and I had instant rapport, and I thought the quiet little town a paradise. After telegraphing the good news to Jill, Pieter and I drove on happily down the coast and into the Blue Mountains, every prospect pleasing, fascinating and exotic.

We left Goondiwindi on a high note, coinciding with the annual garden fete held in the hospital grounds. The town band played selected tunes from light opera, with Johnnie accompanying them silently on his toy trumpet. Teams of marching girls, from kindergarten to young adult-size, paraded competently in brightly coloured tunics. Small children displayed their pets, cats, dogs and goldfish, and we were asked to guess a piglet's weight. The younger nurses presented a fashion show in the latest woollen garments, whilst the middle aged and more mature ladies looked splendid in the latest styles, hats and of course, gloves. After the presentation of prizes, the hospital chairman and members of the shire council asked me to accept a crystal vase and a doctor's bag in appreciation of my two years as hospital doctor.

The ABC radio had a "Hospital Half Hour" program for requests throughout Australia, and had been persuaded to feature Goondiwindi on that day, with martial and farewell music for its departing medical superintendent. So I left to the sounds of the Mounties' chorus, "Goodbye, goodbye, it's time to say goodbye" and some Gilbert and Sullivan.

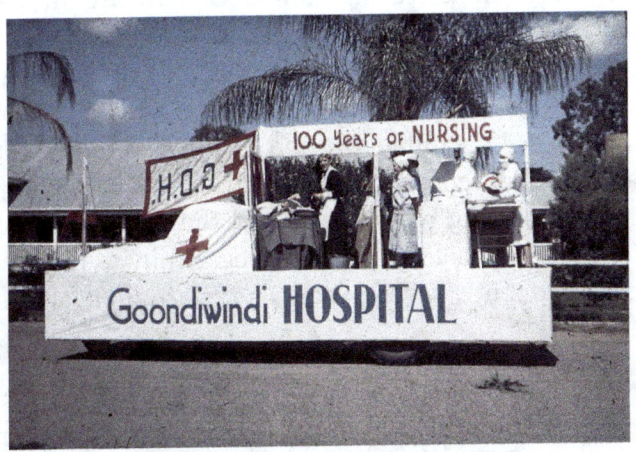

Hopsital float - Goondiwindi parade, 1959

Chapter 12: FAMILY DOCTOR -1

Dr. Macdonald had organised a rented house near the hospital overlooking the southern beaches and the airport. Twice a day, as we were on the direct landing flight path, the commercial flights from Sydney skimmed over our roof, as well as an increasing number of light aircraft making their way along the coast. At the age of two and a half, John was fascinated and explained it, with his chubby finger pointing excitedly as the Airspeed "Elizabethan" floated overhead, as "Ver cum lam", meaning "the aeroplane is coming to land". He later became an air traffic controller in Brisbane. Jill's mother was staying with us and had the pleasure of seeing Rick's first steps, before returning regretfully to England, to return permanently several years later, with Jill's father.

In the early days, the grandparents enjoyed baby sitting for John and Rick. Jill's father had been doing research in England into ancient metrology, studying and measuring the pre-Roman tracks or lays which criss-crossed the West Country. He explored ancient Aboriginal bora grounds and stone piles in the hills near Coffs Harbour and mapped them, suggesting they may have been part of a celestial observatory system. He rented a cottage in the mountains near Ebor to write his findings in peace. He died after having spent a happy nine years, apart from the last year, when Parkinson's disease took its toll. Jill's mother outlived him by two years, dying of breast cancer, so we were able to repay their kindness over the years, by caring for them during their last months.

I spent the first six months as an assistant on a fixed salary. Dr. Mac and I were compatible, so I became a partner, buying in over three years for 50% of a year's income. This was the standard method of entering a practice, the price being for "goodwill" for the number of patients which the senior partner had built up over the years. There were five doctors in Coffs Harbour in 1961 for about seven thousand population. We had a forty bed hospital, originally twelve beds built in 1917, and gradually expanded in a desultory fashion as funds became available. There was local antagonism to fund-raising during this phase, because earlier, £10,000, a very large sum in those days, raised locally for the hospital had ended up in the state coffers for New South Wales, and never reached its rightful destination.

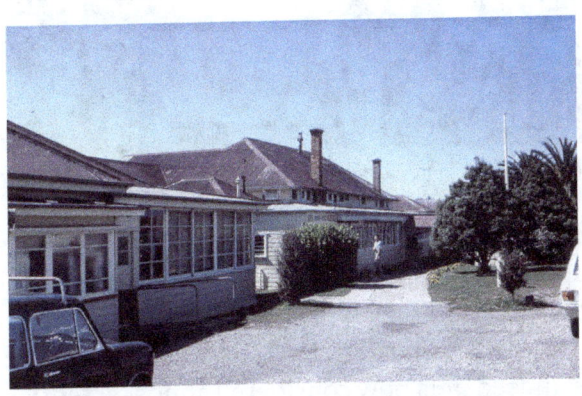

Entrance to the old hospital.

The maternity hospital was a large and rambling private house, Sunnyside, two miles away from the main facilities. It had no sewerage and made use of the dunny-can man, who carted all the waste products off. The lying-in room, with mothers in early labour, was separated from the main labour ward by a very thin wooden wall, through which every moan, scream and cry of encouragement could be heard. Emergency Caesars and forceps cases had to be taken by ambulance to the main hospital. Aboriginal women were delivered in the main hospital on the covered-in balcony of the female ward sometimes separated by only a curtain from a post-operative appendix patient. This pernicious practice ceased shortly after I arrived when the new brick maternity unit attached to the general hospital was opened for all mothers.

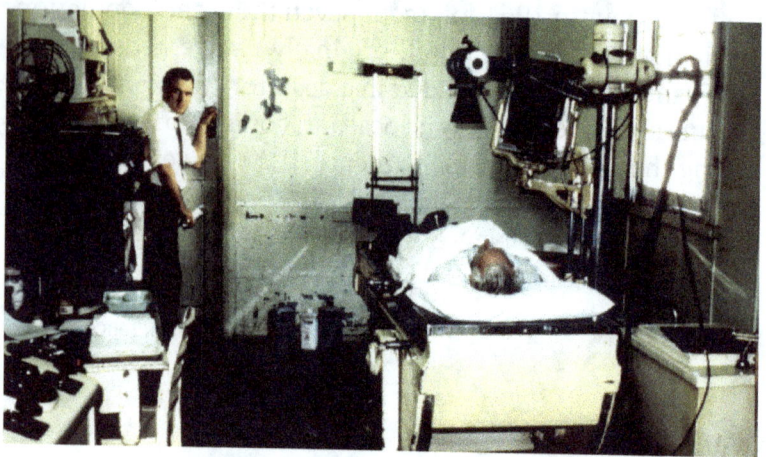

Tony Arnoldus in the X-ray department, 1965

There was still an exclusion of all males except the doctor from the labour ward. When one of our dentists wanted to be with his wife for the delivery, he was allowed to peep through the small window in the door. These rigid rules have long since gone, indeed, it is now considered almost essential for the partner to be present. This is fine with normal births, but can be very traumatic for the attendant in complicated conditions, when interventional obstetrics such as a forceps delivery is essential for the baby's survival. This anxiety can be transferred to the doctor and no doctor likes non-medical surveillance during procedures.

The main hospital had two "public" wards, with the balconies walled in for extra bed space, a childrens' ward, six single "private" rooms, and an eight bedded "intermediate" ward for those patients who were partially covered by insurance. The doctors charged no fees for the public patients, in return for which they were allowed to use the hospital for their private patients. The standard of medical and nursing care was the same, the difference, as nowadays, being in privacy. There was an X-ray unit with a elderly machine and a more elderly radiographer, who had been a wardsman sent away for training. A radiologist drove in from Grafton once weekly to do specialised examinations, such as Barium meals and enemata.

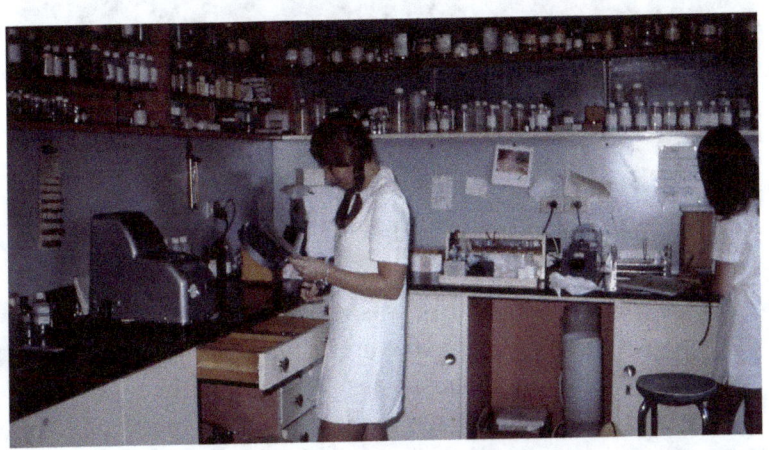

Pathology laboratory, 1965

The operating theatre was small and basic, but had a reasonable array of surgical instruments. The anaesthetics were unsophisticated, relying mostly on ether, a safe mode with the disadvantages of being unusable with diathermy in case of an explosion, and giving headache and nausea on recovery. For operations on the mouth and throat such as tonsillectomy, anaesthesia was by ether dropped onto an electrically heated plate in a glass container. A small pump then passed air over the vapour down a tube into the patient's mouth gag. The depth of anaesthesia was gauged by watching the pupil size, and controlled by the number of drops of ether sizzling on the hot plate.

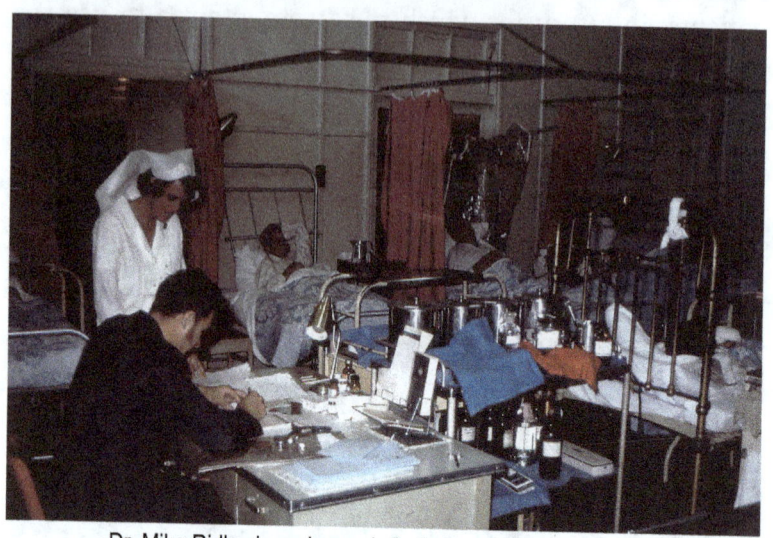

Dr. Mike Ridley in male ward, Coffs Harbour Hospital, 1965

Later we were told this was electrically dangerous and the apparatus sat on a hot water container which rapidly cooled, making anaesthesia less accurate. The surgeon, leaning over the patient's mouth, received a blast of ether vapour, and became quite unsteady during long cases. Three cases were the maximum before the surgeon himself became anaesthetised. Open ether anaesthesia was one of the last arts of medicine, making way for the present scientific, accurate and far safer methods of muscle relaxants and monitoring. Glancing at the pupil size is not possible under the tubes and drapes covering the patient's head. In any case, the muscle relaxant fixes the pupil size. In good hands, ether was a very safe anaesthetic, as the respirations stopped well before the heart if too much was administered. A few squeezes on the chest would blow out the excess and the operation could proceed.

A tiny room near the front entrance doubled as a physiotherapy unit with a staff of one, and as a minor operating theatre. A small laboratory at the driveway entrance allowed us to do basic pathology with the help of two technicians. At first, we had to do all the blood grouping and cross-matching ourselves from a donor panel, as in Goondiwindi. More complicated tests were sent to the nearest qualified pathologist who lived in Grafton, fifty miles away.

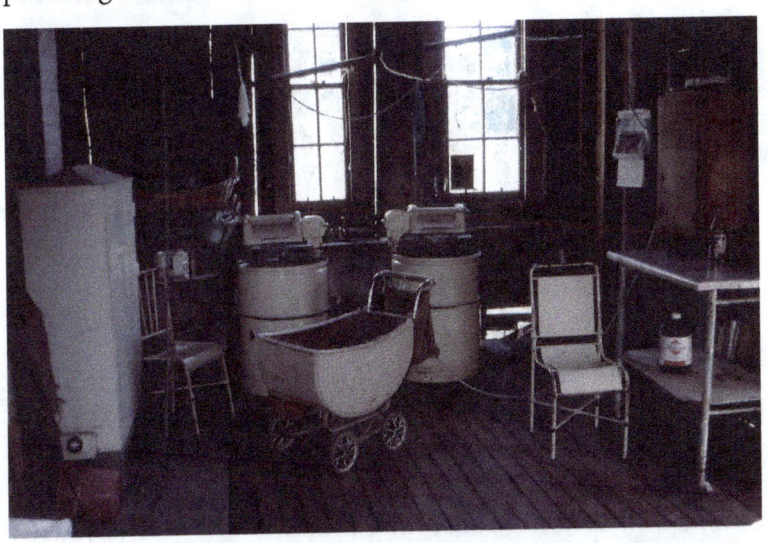

Old Coffs Harbour Hospital laundry, 1965

The administrative staff consisted of the hospital secretary, a chief clerk and a typist. There was a dedicated group of nurses, headed by an able ex-Army Matron. Many had been locally trained as Nurses' Aides and they all wore veils, the traditional Florence Nightingale head gear. The high technology revolution had not yet arrived, and intravenous drips were simple arrangements, to be watched and adjusted frequently. There was one three-channel electrocardiograph and no defibrillator. We had heard of acute and intensive care wards in major city hospitals, but our little hospital had to do its best with expert nursing, oxygen and a limited number of drugs .

The opening of the new four storey brick hospital in 1970 was attended in perfect weather by a brightly dressed crowd sitting outside under parasols. Speeches were made by everyone who was associated with the planning, which had taken twenty five years to bring to fruition, and the Minister of Health unveiled a plaque to commemorate the event. Unfortunately, the printer of the invitation cards had reversed the Q so that it read, "The Minister will then unveil a plague to commemorate the event", hinting at our later troubles from insufficient beds. We had told the Health Department that it was already too small, but were advised to take it or leave it. The same Minister forgot to register in time for the next election and passed into political oblivion.

A typical day's work started with a ward round of the inpatients until about 10 a.m. On operating days, most of the morning was spent in the theatre. I spent the rest of the day seeing those patients who came to our rooms which had been built by Dr. Macdonald opposite his house where he had had his original consulting room. It was very advanced for its day, with three doctors' rooms, each with separate examination annexes, and a minor procedures room, as well as a large waiting room. A quiet back room enabled us to escape for a cup of coffee without running the gauntlet of the accusing eyes of patients waiting not so patiently. It was here, and in a similar tea-room in the hospital that we undertook that very important part of ongoing medical education, the exchange of news and views.

Years later, the pharmaceutical firms began the practice of sponsoring evening talks by specialists in the rapidly expanding fields of medicine. Although they used the opportunity to remind us of their very competitive products with discrete displays, samples and ballpoint pens, the lecturers were for the most part non-partisan and honest in their opinions of these products.

We had these meetings after excellent dinners in one of the larger tourist resorts, until it was realised that we were too sleepy by 9 pm to absorb much information. When the talk became the first item, most of us were too hungry by the time it had finished, especially when the question time was prolonged by personal anecdotes from the audience. A compromise was reached and the lectures were then slotted in between the entrée and the main course.

Once a month, Dr Macdonald, myself, our Nursing Sister and secretary would have a session with the accounts. We would go through the pile of bills, concentrating on the overdue or slow payers. Rainy's previous partner had a simple system of categorising each patient.

A meant an excellent income,

B meant a reasonable income and

C meant very little income.

+ meant a good payer, whilst - meant a poor payer.

Living in a close community, Rainy was well aware of most people's incomes, and many C bills were quietly dropped. A+ cases were welcome but we objected to the A- who ignored repeat accounts and these were the only ones he sent to the debt-collecting agency. Strangely enough, they always came back without animosity for more treatment or opinions. I suppose that their wealth was related to their ability to ignore bill payment until the very last moment.

Home visits, or house-calls are an important part of a country practice. I would check that the batteries for the auriscope functioned and load up my black bag with syringes, blood pressure machine, stethoscope and a few essential medications. I used 1/1000 adrenaline for acute asthma attacks especially when there was clear winter weather and a temperature inversion occurred. A cloud of cold air contaminated with smoke from wood fires, and assorted pollens settled over Coffs Harbour triggering off susceptible bronchial tubes into severe spasm. I used the old pre-metric formula, giving five minims subcutaneously at once, then a minim a minute, converting to metric measures for the later syringes which were marked in millilitres only. Sometimes, I used adrenaline for acute allergic reactions to such foods as tinned peaches or prawns, when the patient was in acute respiratory distress or had a swollen throat or a widespread itchy rash.

Morphia and pethidine, their use carefully recorded in a narcotics register, were the commonest items in a doctor's bag. Nothing beats morphia for the severe pain of a heart attack, and can break the vicious cycle of pain causing more coronary spasm and more pain. An injection can convert a patient at death's door with acutely waterlogged lungs from heart failure, to a cheerful and in no way breathless person whose request for hospital admission is then questioned by the admitting casualty doctor.

Pethidine was the mainstay of treatment of pain associated with violent spasm of internal tubular structures such as the passage of stones from the gall bladder or kidney. But it is also a common request of addicts, who will present with classical symptoms and a tattered letter of doubtful authenticity from a city doctor on a Friday after surgery hours and therefore uncheckable. Some addicts could dislocate their own shoulders and demand pethidine by injection, and then relaxed their muscles sufficiently to allow the shoulder to slip back into position. The only ward using pethidine now is maternity, where addiction would be incredibly unlikely.

Sedatives were all barbiturates, and I carried ampoules of soluble phenobarbitone for epilepsy, and a few capsules of Carbrital or Seconal for those who needed their sleep. These were phased out when the benzodiazepine group became popular as non-addictable sedatives, and Valium was used with effect for epileptics and acute anxiety states. Unfortunately, they did not live up to their original benign promise, and there are just as many patients dependent on them as were on barbiturates.

The main advantage is that overdose is far less lethal. The first phenothiazine, Largactil, had just appeared and was used for psychotic episodes, and Stemetil for nausea and vertigo. At first, acute oedema from cardiac failure was treated with a mercurial diuretic, Neptal or Mersalyl which partially poisoned the kidneys, but the advent of thiazides and frusemide with no deleterious effects on the kidney have made it redundant. The only other injection I carried was penicillin. The syringes were all glass and reusable after boiling. The plastic single-use syringe appeared later, a great time saver, but the huge number produced and careless disposal by addicts have made them a menace to cleaners and members of the public, risking needle stick injury, hepatitis and AIDS.

After a couple of years as partner, I decided to go to Melbourne for a refresher course in surgery and have an attempt at the final surgical fellowship examination. We contacted an English doctor who was emigrating to

Australia, as a *locum tenens*, and I met him in Sydney the day his ship docked. He seemed a cheery sort of person, his red nose showing he had obviously enjoyed the sunshine on the voyage out. I took him to lunch at the old Metropole hotel, and offered him wine, warning him of the high incidence of alcoholics in his new country. He and his lady friend set up in the flat above the consulting rooms, where they had frequent noisy arguments and drinking parties. He used my car which he drove into a ditch, or parked every day outside Sawtell Returned Servicemen's Club. Our surgery Sister had to walk loudly down to his room to give him time to put his bottle away. He was asked to leave after attempting to stitch one side of a wound only. He went on to Papua-New Guinea where he later died of liver failure. It compromised my three month course, but Rainy insisted I finish it.

In my second year of general practice, a small, very active American called in with a minor ailment. John Landi was an entomologist who was searching for natural predators of parasitic scale insects, for the Californian Sunkist orange company. We became good friends after he decided to stay in Coffs Harbour, having seen the potential of a banana plantation a little north of the town on the Pacific Highway. He decided to pull down the derelict packing shed by the turn in the road, and build the Biggest Banana in the World. A local engineer scaled up plans from a genuine banana. It was made from concrete over chicken wire with a passageway containing large pictures showing the various aspects of the banana industry, packing, cutting, trashing (cutting off the old dead leaves), de-suckering, fertilising, bagging and putting up supportive wooden props. He then made a pathway to a small observation post, the Tiki Hut, overlooking the bay.

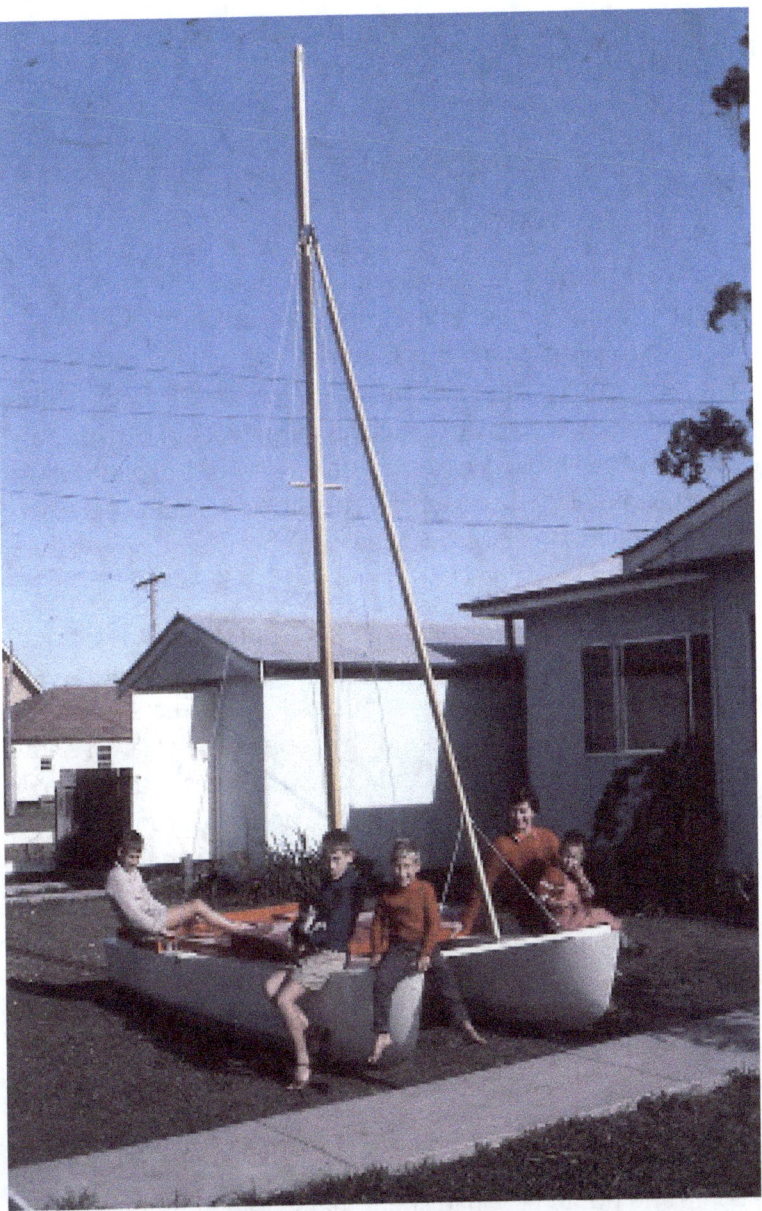

Jill and the four boys on 'Echo', our homebuilt catameran, 1964

I would occasionally take sightseers around the plantation and explain what hard work bananas are. I also enjoyed people's reactions to little jokes.

"Why do you put blue bags over the bunches?" was a common question.

"Well," I would say, "Bananas mate at night and if you keep them dark, you get bigger bunches." The real reason is that the hot house effect produces bigger bananas, and small squares of pest strip material are nailed to the stem making a microclimate of insecticide, as well as providing some protection from the ravages of parrots and fruit bats. If the visitors looked extra gullible, I would explain about the multiple bladed scissors to cut the leaves and the way of recognising a banana grower by one short leg from walking on the hillside all day.

Jill and I had tried to take a break from work at least once a year. We were forty-three years old and enjoying two weeks in summer in the Snowy Mountains. Out of the ski season, Thredbo village was quiet and the mountains clear of snow, replaced by alpine flowers and clear streams chortling down to join the river in the valley below. The ski-lift took us to the granite outcrop overlooking the chalets and hotels. We took deep breaths of mountain air and, free from worries, strolled, walked and gambolled downhill, through heather meadows, clumps of gnarled alpine trees, crossing and recrossing a crystal brook. We each carried a bag containing cold drinks and chocolate bars slung over our shoulders. That evening, Jill told me she felt a lump in her breast. It was an early cancer.

I felt totally shaken. These things happened to other people and not to us. I had spent many hours talking sensibly to women about the options available, and cautiously optimistically to their husbands, encouraging them to give all the support they could to their wives. I had seen the terrible anxious look on their faces but had not until then, realised the state of mind they were in.

Breast cancer, although so common, appears when least expected. Routine mammography came with the next decade and has halved the mortality rate.

I contacted Harry Cumberland, a Sydney surgeon, and we drove down, myself subdued and trying to keep my face away from Jill in the car, so she would not see the trickle of tears. I had too much knowledge of the possibilities, especially in her age group. She had steeled herself and faced the prospect of surgery bravely. We stayed at our old Goondiwindi friend Tom's Sydney house, with his wife Betty giving Jill encouragement. Two days later, I left her at the hospital and, rather than sit around, I walked endlessly along Sydney streets for three hours.

The operation was a success and Jill returned to Coffs Harbour four weeks later. Jill's brother Tony was in Australia at the time and I met him at Sydney Airport, where, seeing in his face Jill's blue eyes, I made a fool of myself by openly weeping in the lounge, much to Tony's embarrassment. Fifteen years later, she had another cancer on the other side, again successfully removed. I can identify with similar patients and their family members and know exactly what they are going through, but as Jill has already survived for over twenty-five years, I can be very encouraging to new cases I have seen.

CHAPTER 13: FLYING

I had completed my flying licence in a Cessna 150 flown up every two weeks from Port Macquarie, half an hour away. A policemen who had an instructor's rating was appointed to the local police station, so a small group of aircraft enthusiasts decided to resurrect the old Coffs Harbour Aero Club. We bought an old but reliable Tiger Moth and I was elected president. Within a few months, the club had expanded and added two more modern Cessnas to its fleet.

A chance visit to an ambulance driver at Macksville who was constructing a single-seater Jodel D-9 aircraft, set me on the path to home-building a two-seater version, a D-11. It was made in my carport and garden shed from aircraft grade spruce and plywood, glued together with resorcinol resin, covered with Irish linen fabric sewn over the wing ribs with waxed thread, and finally painted with dope. Half finished pieces were stored around the bedroom, under the bed and behind the settee in the lounge, with minimal protests from Jill.

The first engine I used had been on the original Australian built wooden Victa monoplane. The 65 hp provided too little power for its high wing loading, but was ideal for the slow, high lift wing of the Jodel. I changed it for a 100 hp

Continental later, to have better performance and a generator for the radio.

It was carefully examined at progressive stages by the two Freds, Civil Aviation Department inspectors, helpful and sympathetic to a newcomer. They were a fountain of aeronautical safety lore, and had been involved in numerous accident investigations. They advised me to turn the battery around, to prevent sparking in the event of a crash, and to put the balance weight under the tail, not inside the fuselage, as a pilot had once been killed by the loosened lump of steel flicking forward in a crash. Sitting on the lounge settee after we had been doing the carbon monoxide flight tests, the non-smoking Fred said to Fred the smoker, "breath out", and took a sample of his exhaled smoke. It contained ten times the level allowable in an aircraft in flight.

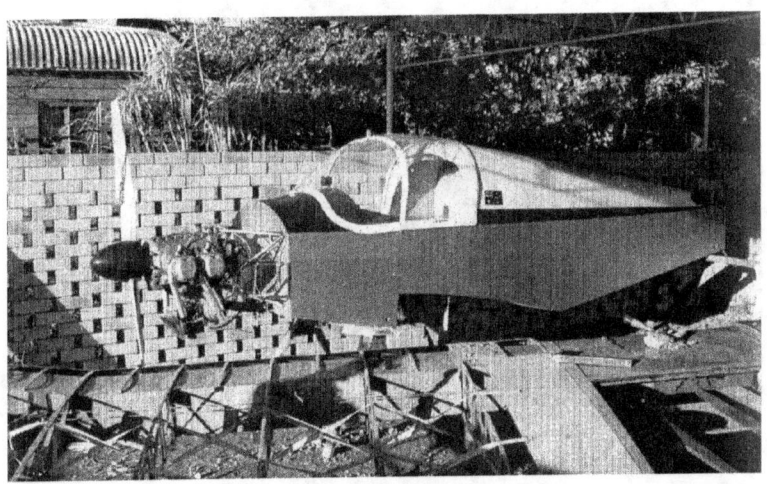

Building the Jodel in the carport, 1967

I had to glue sample scraps of wood with each batch of resorcinol adhesive, and the wood, not the glue, had to break first under stress. All metal welding had to be done by a certified expert, and all nuts and bolts were of aircraft quality and there-fore four times the cost of hardware store articles. I painted her in BOAC colours, with a feather-tailed glider, the smallest flying possum, on the rudder, and secured the registration letters VHDRJ, Delta Romeo Juliet.

Two years after buying the plans, she was finished, and I was allowed to test fly her. The first flight was faultless, and was one of the high spots of my life, floating sedately over Coffs Harbour, with an enormous smile on my face. I had been helped by a neighbour, recently arrived from Nowra, Newton Lawson, who was also building a very similar type. My other neighbour, Lou Simmons, also a pilot, decided to build another Jodel D-11, and eventually, there were three light aircraft built in adjoining suburban houses, which must be a record.

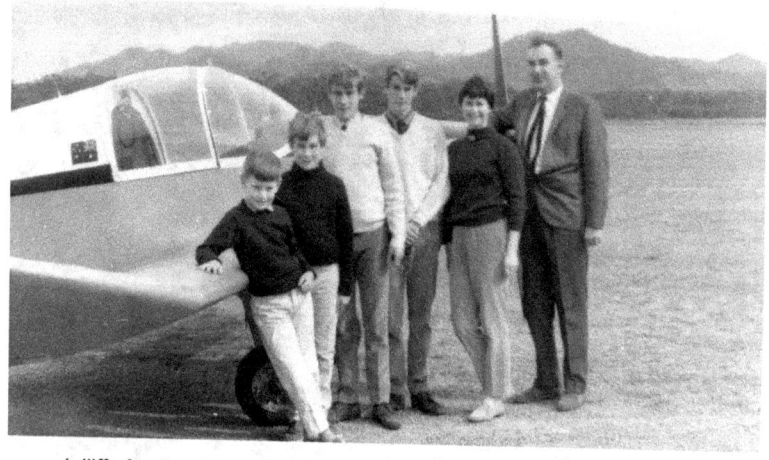

Jelliffe family with Jodel, 1969: Rick, John, Peter, Michael, Jill & Robin

I flew my delightful plane for over 800 hours, over the Barrier Reef, down to Melbourne, and on several air races. The races all involved flying for more than a thousand miles over two days, with an overnight stop in a small Western town. After anxiously checking the weather map on TV the previous evening, aircrew for over 150 competing aircraft gathered before dawn in a bitterly cold hangar, as the races were usually held during the less turbulent winter months, ostensibly in better weather. Rugged up and shivering, some yawning with hangovers from the pre-race parties, the pilots listened carefully to the briefing officer whose main concern was to see the affair completed without casualties.

There were usually four intermediate stops, and the planes were handicapped from their known cruising speed and fuel consumption. Any "throttle-bending" would be obvious by the excess amount of fuel used, being worked out by the amount needed to refill the tanks. We gave a final inspection, checked the oil level, the fuel tank for water condensation, waggled the controls and we were ready.

We took off at maximum all-up-weight, and I had to put sandbags in the luggage compartment as my navigators were usually light persons. All navigation was by dead reckoning and the electronic instruments were sealed off, leaving the compass alone. As my Jodel had no such luxuries, I was at an advantage. I was used to finding my way across long distances with watch and compass alone, looking out of the windscreen at the topography as it corresponded with the map. We soon found it was dangerous to follow another aircraft, as many of them were wildly off course. We identified mountain tops, railways, roads and towns as they came up on-schedule, and chose our height by the predicted winds, aiming to collect a tail wind component. As much of the flying was over miles of hot, dry scrub country with thermals in the shape of swirling dust-devils rising as high as 8,000 feet at midday, we flew as high as possible, but were still tossed about in our light craft. It was always a relief to see our last destination for the day ahead. Suddenly, having seen no other aircraft for hours, we were surrounded by our competitors arriving and anxious to cross the finishing line on time, often from odd directions which showed how lost some of them had been.

Often, we were given beds on the large open balcony of a country hotel. Some bright young men would keep talking after a beer or two, to everybody's irritation, until a burly voice would sound. "Keep quiet, or I'll come and belt you." Another unwelcome prank was to wake us all two hours too early with the announcement that it was briefing time. When we did arrive for briefing, most of us felt we had not had our fair share of rest.

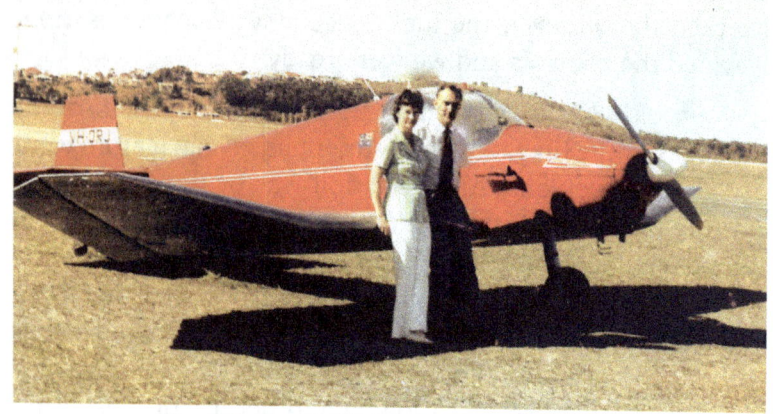

Jill and Robin with VH-DRJ in later colour scheme

After final arrival, our planes were inspected and given a last top-up of petrol to ensure that we had used the genuine cruise rate, and we were ready to hear the race results in different categories. I once won one of the six race legs and accepted my prize from the then Premier of Queensland. During that race, we had suddenly flown into a layer of very cold air. Lou, my little navigator, suddenly tucked his legs up under him and and said, "I've gotta pee!" He managed to hold off till the next stop, but leapt out of the plane before it had stopped, to relieve himself in the shadow of the wing, shielded from the welcoming crowd by the broad side of the fuselage. I introduced him as the only navigator on whom you had to do a pre-flight water test as well as in the fuel.

Lou would fly alongside me in his own Jodel around the Coffs Harbour area where we would formate on the Tiger Moth, the nearest I ever felt to the World War I dawn patrols. I landed on the beach on many occasions, on the firm sand between the tide marks, and followed the rivers and roads up into the mountains over thickly forested "tiger" country, with no chance of a forced landing if the engine failed. Two of my sons used the plane to gain flying hours for their pilot licences, and I lent it on several occasions, sometimes with disastrous results.

An improperly fastened canopy blew open and smashed the perspex, and an unauthorised adjustment to the rudder controls caused a ground loop and bent propeller. The usual answer was "Sorry", and little else. My plane, I decided, should be like pen and wife, not to be lent. I sold it after twelve years of delightful flying to help with some educational needs, and it is still flying in Western Australia, nearly forty years old.

Lou decided to make a faster aircraft, and chose a mini-Mustang, a metal two-seater with a larger engine and a speed of 135 knots, as against the Jodel's 95 knots. We built it together, mostly in his ice factory, over six years. Neither of us had any experience with metal, yet we managed to rivet the complex structure without a blemish, to produce a streamlined fighterlike machine of classic lines. We knew that the Civil Aviation inspectors could never pass any work as perfect, so we left one rivet in the fuselage in an easily accessible place in a partially compressed state. They found it, congratulated us on an otherwise excellent job and we then completed the rivet in question.

A few years later, at the age of fifty five, I had my final urge to construct another flying machine, this time in fibreglass, carbon fibre, foam and epoxy resin. I chose an unusual shape, a tandem two-seater biplane, called a "Dragonfly", with a front low wing and a shoulder wing midway along the fuselage, but no horizontal tail plane. It was powered by a converted 2100 Volkswagen engine. The original design had the wheels at the front wing tips, (as illustrated on the front cover) but this proved very tricky to land and I later changed it to a more conventional configuration. It took two years to build and was delightful to fly, but was potentially dangerous to land. The propeller was close to the ground, and the front wing had a habit of pitching down at the critical touchdown speed. Once, three feet above the runway, she wiped off the wheels.

I cut my losses, sold the engine and replaced it with a spindle under the cowling attached to an unairworthy propellor. I replaced the radio and instruments with photographs, sold the originals and donated the air frame to Wangaratta Air Museum, with instructions that it should never be flown again. For a while it hung safely from the hangar roof, keeping company with fifty other interesting planes. I had it for five years and 100 hours flying. I can sleep easily, knowing that no-one will kill themselves in my aircraft. An expensive exercise, to paraphrase the definition usually made about boats, "An aircraft is a hole in the sky into which one pours money".

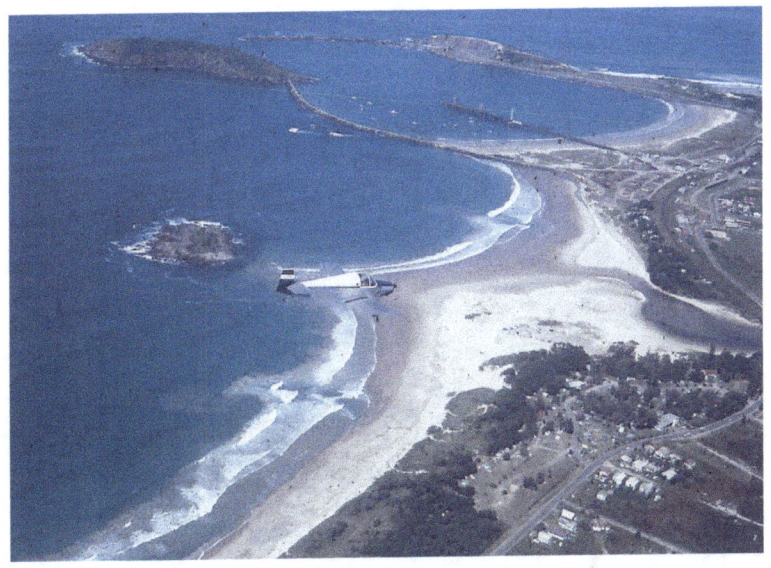

Jodel D-11 VH-DRJ in original colours over Coffs Harbour, 1968

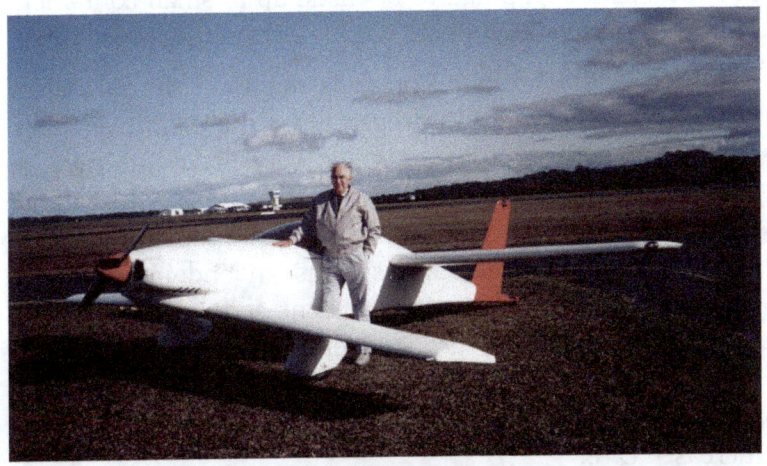

Dragonfly with modified undercarriage, 1994

CHAPTER 14: NEW GUINEA INTERLUDES

Soon after building the two-seater Jodel aircraft, I joined Coffs Harbour Rotary Club, and in 1968, went to Wasu on the north coast of the Territory of Papua & New Guinea[2] (TPNG) as part of a team building a wharf. Up till then, all produce had been rowed ashore from the coastal freighter standing outside the coral reefs at considerable risk of spoiling from salt water, or even total loss in rough weather. The local coffee crop had to be made up in small containers to fit the equally small boats, a time-consuming procedure.

Twelve Coffs Harbour Rotarians made up the second of three teams. We were ill-prepared for the primitive living conditions, little ground tents and very little anti-malarial precautions. The party had unjustified faith in anti-malarial medication, not realising that this part of the world which looked like a tropical Paradise was an endemic area for resistant strains of the most virulent and potentially fatal type. Ten out of our group eventually went down with malarial attacks on returning to Australia. I was one of the lucky two, perhaps because of my Nigerian experience and increased care.

About a third of the wharf had been completed and each member of the team had jobs according to their ability. The only experience I had was with welding, but they already had a professional for the one welding machine. After welding, the large steel tubular pipes were coated with thick bitumen paint and then driven into the coral with a pile driver. The process was made more exciting by the deafness of the man holding the pipes. Once, the welding machine contacted the sea where the welder was standing and only quick action shutting off the generator saved us from a fatality. As the superstructure progressed seawards, wooden sleepers were laid on top, accompanied by uncontrollable laughter from the New Guinean helpers. This was due to a subtle language difference. We had been shouting "push, push" (as *'pushim'*), which refers to sexual intercourse in Pidgin English. The word should have been "shove" (*subim* in Pidgin).

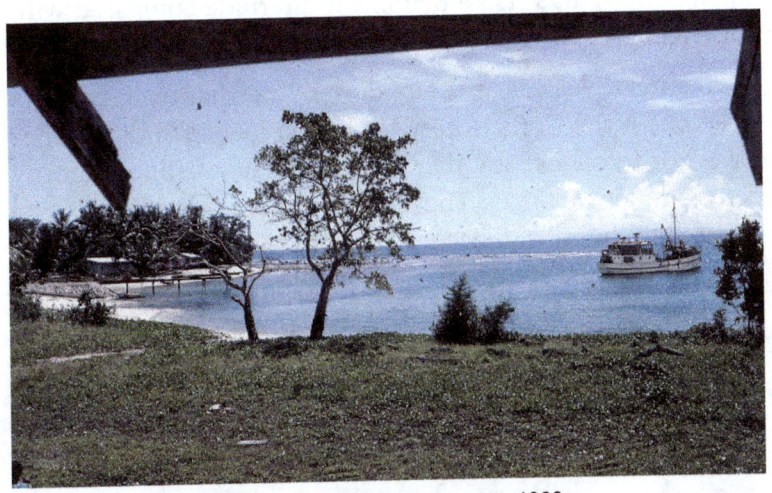

Wasu wharf, TPNG north coast, 1968

John Landi, my Big Banana friend and I found ourselves superfluous, and heard that a Sister Maria Horne in the Lutheran leprosy hospital in the mountains needed help with concreting and covering pathways between the sleeping quarters.

We transferred up through exquisitely beautiful slopes to Etep at 3,000 feet with a view out over the whole northern New Guinea coast, the sea clouds accentuating the row of volcanic islands and emerald beaches fringed with white coral. At last we were truly in paradise. We had comfortable beds, virtually no mosquitoes and a superb climate.

In late afternoon, after completing our day's concreting using crushed sea shells for lime, the cloud layer crept uphill and we heard the patter of raindrops ending in a short downpour. The evening mist rolled magically in and hundreds of fireflies flickered through the forest. At the end of our stay, the patients put on a sing-sing for us, with fantastic high head gear decorated with vines and flowers, to say thanks for our work. We had had a delightful interlude compared with our friends' relative misery at the hot and humid wharf site.

The next year, I was appointed international projects director for the Coffs Rotary Club, and met with the district governor to choose another project in New Guinea, shortly before independence. The Asia Pacific Christian Mission wished to build a teacher training college at Dauli near Tari, in a rather remote region of the Southern Highlands Province, away from disruptive tribal influences, to which different language groups could safely come. Over one hundred trainee teachers would start the courses, increasing with time. Our job was to supply expertise with the building, but first we had to make a feasibility study.

Armed with twenty packs of 8 mm movie film to make a record for later recruitment of workers, we set off in a locally owned twin-engined Beechcraft Baron aircraft. Jill, myself, three local Rotarians and the pilot flew up to Tari, a two day trip by dead reckoning, arriving through a gap in the otherwise solid cloud cover. We spent five days as the missionaries' guests in the land of the Huli warriors, which had seen its first white exploration only thirty-five years before. Its first district officer had to contend with murderous tribal fights, and there had been a pay-back killing with the victim skewered by arrows only three years previously.

We were supposed to be assessing the missionaries and their plan for further education of the New Guineans, but I had the feeling that they were assessing us to see if we were serious and not just a group of bumbling do-gooders. Each side fulfilled the other's criteria and the project was confirmed.

Back in Coffs Harbour, we formed up a committee to set the project in motion, but eventually it was easier to arrange it by myself. Firstly, I had to find volunteers and put an article in the Rotary journal with a photograph of a Huli man in his brightly coloured wig decorated with birds of paradise feathers. The project was called "Operation Big-wig". I used my aircraft to visit several reasonably close Rotary clubs and showed the film I had put together which encouraged many to consider joining.

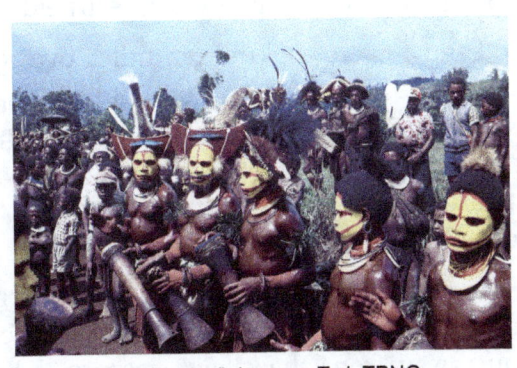

Huli "singsing" dancers, Tari, TPNG

The recompense for staying overnight in a strange bed was flying back at crack of dawn in silky smooth air over the mountains, and seeing the sun arising out of the Pacific Ocean, outlining the Solitary Islands as I approached Coffs Harbour.

My study was a pre-computer age mess of papers, charts, application forms and correspondence with missionaries, airlines, and volunteers, some from as far away as America. I was determined the exercise should be efficiently, comfortably and safely run. Sixty-five volunteers finally made their decision and paid me the fixed airline fare and the charter flights into Tari, totalling $250. The final tally showed us to be $4 each down, due to a charter plane turning back with bad weather, not a bad estimate.

We were in three main groups of twenty each, aged mostly in our thirties and forties, flying up at fortnightly intervals to Mount Hagen where we stayed overnight with Rotarian families before taking the hour's flight by light aircraft to Tari. There were several wives who were invaluable in the "hotel" arrangements in our huts. Jim Erkkila, a tough missionary who had walked into Tari years before and who spoke fluent Huli, met us at the airfield.

Land Rovers took us ten miles over glassy slippery clay roads to the training college site, sliding sideways, wheels spinning in deep potholes and requiring all hands to push them up steep inclines. A team of missionary carpenters had already started work and had completed the dining hut and dormitories.

In my applications form, I had asked for snorers to confess their nocturnal noises, and they were housed in a separate hut away from the silent sleepers. I had had experience of holidays spoilt by sleepless noisy nights and resultant drooping days.

After years of negotiating with the multiple land owners, the Asia Pacific Christian Mission had acquired a stand of hoop pine, tall, straight and easy to work without seasoning. A group of friendly and enthusiastic Huli men stood on the trees as soon as they were felled and stripped the bark off with precise axe cuts. My favourite was a small man with a cheerful charming manner who had five payback killings to his name. At first the timber was cut into planks by pit saw with one man standing on the log pulling a two-handed saw upwards, whilst his partner, covered with sawdust, stood in a pit pulling it downwards. Later, the Air Force brought in some heavy milling equipment as part of an exercise and a reasonably sized circular saw driven by a Volkswagen engine speeded up the process. At one stage, the timber was felled, milled and put into place on the same day. There was no problem of the hoop pine warping in an environment with such a steady humidity.

We started with the main hall, putting up the tubular steel bearings set in concrete and covered with ant caps to deter the ferocious attacks of white ants, levelling with a theodolite. We laid the open flooring joists and prepared the wall frames at the base of their future positions for easy erection. A mixture of six foot Australians and five foot Hulis then started to lift the heavy framework into the upright position with near disastrous results.

The Hulis stayed together at one end and could not manage to get their end over the critical 60 degrees, and the whole wall began to fall backwards. Most people managed to jump safely between the floor joists, as the uprights fell on either side of them, but one of our volunteers had his chest caught and sustained a fractured rib. Our cook, a man from the lowlands, had severe bruising to his abdomen which I feared could have torn his spleen, which would have been an impossible situation to deal with in our primitive surroundings. He was not a Huli "one-talk", but was from a different tribe, otherwise it could have triggered off possible payback retribution. Luckily his condition improved.

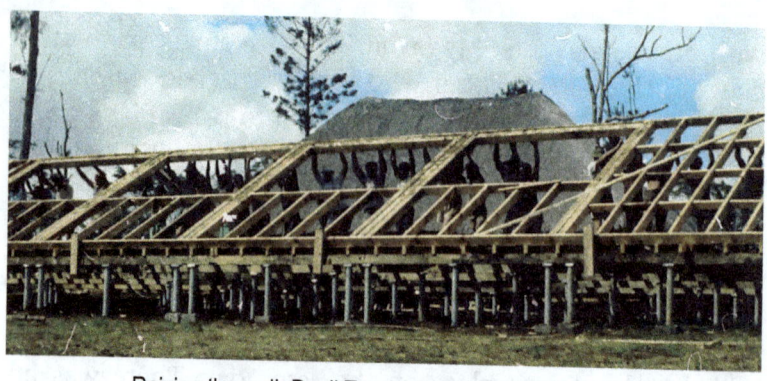
Raising the wall, Dauli Teacher's College, Tari

The Hulis have a second language for carrying messages over long distances by yodelling, and the word went out that we had had a serious accident. Each family group mobilised its warriors and ran down the mountain sides to assess the damage, relaxing their belligerent attitudes when it was found that no Huli had been injured. We knew about the killing of truck drivers who had knocked over pedestrians and had immediately been killed at the road side as payback. I hate to think of our situation if the Hulis had not been small enough to slide nimbly between the floor joists. We tightened up our safety precautions, spreading the Australian contingent evenly amongst the Hulis and attached several safety ropes. There were no more incidents, but our injured volunteer had to be sent home. We had truly become foundation members of Dauli Teacher Training College.

Our most useful members were two plumbers who made water tanks out of corrugated sheets of steel and, even more usefully, taught some of the locals the basics of plumbing and roofing. During the first week, our team nearly finished the main hall and three class rooms. Roy Riddel and I did the easy wall jobs, the noggings, those short pieces of wood which keep the uprights from bowing in. We put up a notice,

"QUALNOGS, Noggings for the Gentry".

When the hall had been walled and floored, the missionaries decided to hold a film night, which was a new experience to many Hulis. Jim Erkkila warned us that we would be unable to talk as all the audience would be shouting and exclaiming at the wonders of the ciné screen. As night fell, flickering lines of torches, hand-held bundles of slow-burning leaves, snaked silently down from the hills. The hall filled up, men on one side and women with children on the other, as in their church. The first film was a documentary showing traffic in Sydney which was really beyond the comprehension of the villagers. Then came the film I had put together during my visit the previous year.

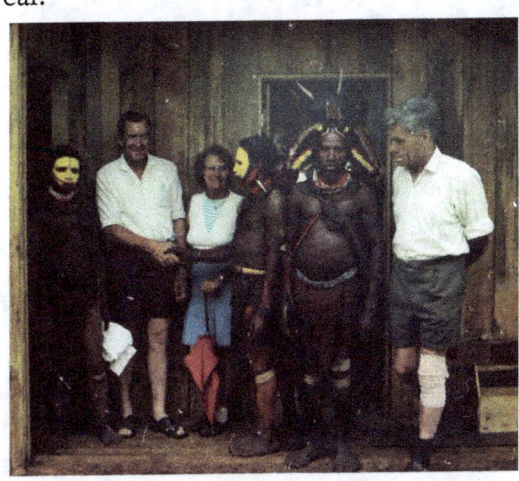

Rotary team meeting Huli's, Tari, 1970

It was one of the most exciting moments of my life. They saw themselves for the first time, and called out when their friends appeared, laughing delightedly, a little confused at their own appearance. Jim was laughing beside me, trying to translate the remarks, including some appreciative ones about the younger womens' topless attributes, which would seem to be a common human trait. We continued hearing them excitedly discussing the evening's entertainment as they left for their long march back over the hills, marked by the line of torches, until they disappeared over the crests.

There was no work on Sundays which we spent sightseeing. We came upon some young men putting on a sing-sing (dance) by a group of houses. Splendidly decorated wigs with bird of paradise feathers topped their lean muscular bodies which they had painted with ochre. Their nasal septa were pierced to accommodate thin bones or feathers and around their necks, they wore pigs' teeth, with a hornbill beak on their backs. Around their waists, they wore kilts of grass or leaves. Known as "arse-grass" these bobbed up and down as they began their dance, to the delight of the assembled and appreciative throng of dowdily dressed women. The dance step was a basic jumping up and down on one spot with a slight sideways progression, to a rapid drum beat for about five minutes, followed by a short rest to allow recovery of their calf muscles, which the women were openly admiring. Close by, a small group of pre-pubertal young girls were dressed up with yellow and red facial make-up and were doing their own little dance holding onto a pole, but these were the only brightly dressed females we saw.

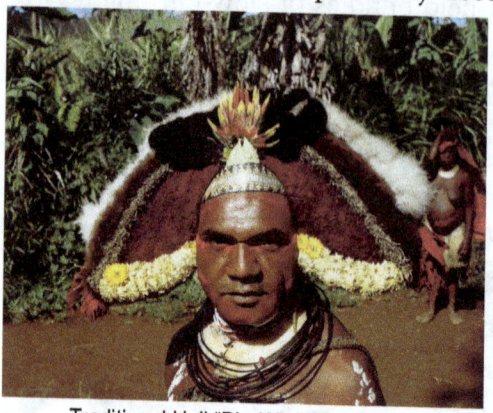
Traditional Huli "Big-Wig", Tari, TPNG

The Huli people lived in damp dark huts, with small smoky fires to keep warm at night and repel mosquitoes. The incidence of malaria was much less than at the coast but conditions such as pneumonia and chronic bronchitis were rife. Often the brighter boys were sent away to the coastal schools, sometimes to face death from cerebral malaria against which they had built up little resistance, as they did not consider malarial prophylaxis necessary.

Leprosy was a scourge and we visited a leprosy village close by, run by the Methodist church. Most of the cases had burnt-out nerve damage, sitting with stubs for fingers and ulcerated toes.

On my first visit to Tari, I had been asked to hold a clinic for the Australian missionaries who had come for their annual conference. One of them had a typical leprosy patch on her forearm which she had been treating with an antifungal ointment. Whether she had deliberately disregarded it, or failed to identify it on a white skin, I never knew.

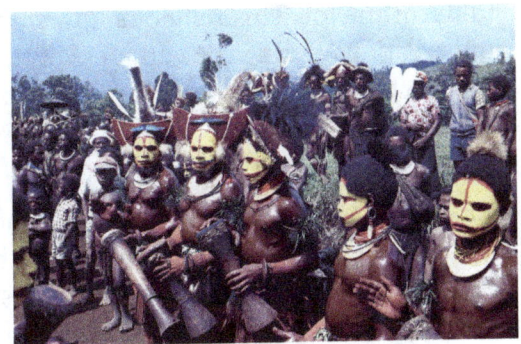

Huli singsing dancers, Tari 1970

At the end of our fortnight, Roy, myself and a Rotary couple hired a car from Mount Hagen and drove extremely carefully down the only road in the highlands to Lae on the north coast. A car had injured a boy playing chicken across a dead end road out of Mt. Hagen, and the locals were known to be waiting vengefully for its return. The owner did a quick respray in a different colour and returned safely.

I had to speak to the Lae Rotary club about our project, apparently successfully, although I can remember very little of the event. The club consisted of toughened old coffee planters and prospectors with a high tolerance to alcohol, higher than mine. The next day, I spoke to the Madang club, and started out in a similar light-hearted tone, until I realised that most of the members were not amused, with a high proportion of missionaries.

I quickly changed my tune. One missionary proudly told me he had returned after the Japanese withdrawal to find that the local people had stored their juju fetish objects in the loft of the church, so he had poured petrol around them and burnt the lot. This religious intolerance reminded me of similar actions during the conquest of the Incas and Mayans when all their records were burnt by the priests as heathen objects.

The next year, the Rotary clubs hired a DC3 aircraft and took some of the original workers and other interested parties to Tari for the official opening of the Teacher Training College. Roy and I joined it at Glen Innes and we droned up the Queensland coast to Port Moresby where we picked up a pilot with the local knowledge needed to fly in the highlands, where the weather is treacherous, the mountains rise up to 15,000 feet and navigational aids are virtually non-existent.

We landed early enough at Tari, but the opening ceremonies were delayed by protocol and the presence of rival Huli warriors, ominously bearing flatbladed war arrows, instead of the usual round-pointed hunting shafts. The speeches were interrupted frequently by loud provocative comments between the adversaries. Jim Erkkila looked anxious as he said that the tempers were at breaking point and soon after, small groups of armed men rushed around the campus, but no clash occurred, and the arrival of yams, pork and chicken meat from the hot stone pit ovens mellowed the situation.

One dignified old man who had recognised me from the work team presented me with a whole half-cooked chicken which I carried around for an hour, uncertain of polite protocol. I appreciated the gesture, and once more Jim Erkkila rescued me by taking it for his group of Hulis. By the time the ceremonies and feasts were over, it was late midday, and the daily cumulus clouds stretched ominously up over the mountains, highly dangerous storm cells which could toss an aircraft upside down and snap its wings off.

When our time to depart Tari came, we took off towards a gap in the clouds which quickly closed. The only way out was obscured and at 10,000 feet we plunged deep into the threatening haze. The elderly Rotarian sitting in behind me clicked his false teeth noisily in direct proportion to the anxiety of the situation, and as we climbed higher and finally up to 15,000 feet, he slumped back with a grey tinge, teeth silent at last. The DC3 is not pressurised and the local pilot called for oxygen for the passengers, which we did not have, neither was it fitted with paddle propellor blades for higher altitudes.

Roy walked happily to the cockpit and announced that ice was across the windscreen, and the pitot head, which measured our all important airspeed, was icing up. Our bright little stewardess had collapsed semi-conscious in her seat, and I had a splitting headache. There was one small handheld oxygen bottle, which the two pilots passed to each other like marijuana joint at a hippy party. Suddenly, we flew out of the side of the cloud into clear blue sky with the north coast beneath us, and quickly descended to a more comfortable altitude. The reassuring sound of clattering false teeth started again behind me, and we landed at Madang with a strong urge to kiss the ground.

The next day, we flew east along the coast to Lae, circling the wharf at Wasu which seemed to be in excellent condition despite the frequent earthquakes in the area. Our DC3 adventures were not quite over. Leaving Mackay, the pilot must have noticed a warning light, and found that the undercarriage would not lock down, but he continued on to Brisbane, after banking steeply to try to wrench the wheels down by G-forces. The clatter of false teeth reached a crescendo, to be cut short by instructions from the stewardess to remove dentures and bend forward in our seats as we landed silently and safely with both engines cut, and were towed ignominiously backwards off the runway.

My next trip to New Guinea was in 1974, with Jill, partly to revisit Etep, Sister Maria Horne, and Michael, now working as a pilot, but mostly to meet Kathy, who took up a large part of his letters home. She is the eldest of six children to Doug and Margaret Parrington, who were stationed at Oro Bay on the coast near Popondetta, working for the Summer Institute of Linguistics (SIL) for several years. Kathy turned out to be a quiet self-reliant young lady who had once canoed down the Sepik river and could set her mind to do anything practical.

Doug's function was to tabulate and clarify the Ewage Notu language of the coastal strip of Oro Bay, Buna and Gona, the landing point of WWII Japanese invasion forces moving to cross the Kokoda Trail. He would spend hours listening to and recording the sounds, and trying to work out a grammar, in this the 100th tribal language for SIL

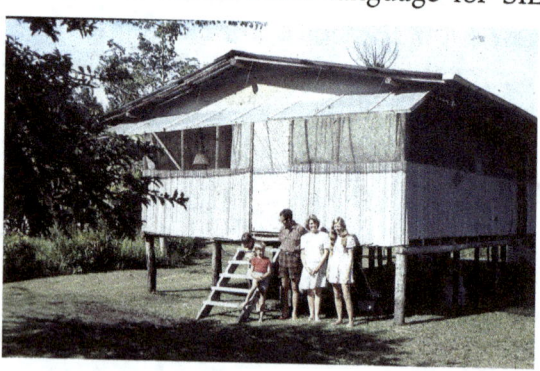

The Parrington's village house at Oro Bay, 1974 (Kathy on right)

in PNG. Every year, all the similar workers would gather at Ukarumpa in the Highlands to compare their results. There are around 800 Melanesian languages, most in PNG, the result of isolated communities, although neighbouring tribes can usually communicate easily. The end result of years of such work was a translation of the New Testament, which was the goal of the missionaries, and a grammar and dictionary of potentially lost languages, the objective of the government. Before he retired, Doug had the satisfaction of completing both.[3]

From Lae, we caught a small coastal trading ship for Wasu. During the day, we sat on the narrow deck watching the bright blue sea, the glaring white sandy shore with its coral fringes and the mountain backdrop, an earthly paradise. But it was a hellish night. The only cabin was an oven-like, narrow claustrophobic space, without ventilation, smelling of oil and old sweat. The tidal surges of the straits of Vitiaz between New Guinea and New Britain rolled us about. The other passengers, all Papua New Guineans, sensibly slept on the open deck under the stars, cooled by the sea breeze. We awoke with headaches and furred tongues in time to disembark onto our famous wharf at Wasu, where we were met by Sister Maria in a four-wheel drive vehicle.

Three thousand feet up at Etep, the lepers gave us a riotous singsing welcome and we felt we were back in paradise. We had a wonderful week. They took us to the extensive caves full of fossilised sea shells, hollowed out in the limestone mountains thrust up by immense geological forces, for New Guinea is the fastest rising island in the world. Some of the patients came with us, laughing and chattering through forest tracks, trim gardens of sweet potatoes with pig enclosures, past huts with trays of drying coffee, to a spectacular waterfall plunging nearly one thousand feet over the edge of the escarpment.

After each return to the organised sophistication of Australia, I had a few days of reverse culture-shock. The consumer-based society, the shallowness of advertising and inane TV programs, were difficult to reconcile with the apparent idylliic life-style I had just left. It was a sobering thought that beneath this beauty, lay the numerous diseases which make life short and unpleasant in the tropics, the killer malaria and the maimer leprosy, and more recently the spread of HIV.

CHAPTER 15: FAMILY DOCTOR - 2

In 1978, we moved from our house in town to a delightful five acre property in a banana growing area five miles south of town, where we built a small but comfortable hexagonal house of western red cedar. We gradually cleared most of the bananas and planted mangoes, litchees and other assorted fruit which are by now very mature. Koalas visit us, the males calling loudly "like a Harley-Davison motor bike on heat" from the surrounding forest. Possums scuttle on the roof, and we host over seventy types of birds. Dawn is heralded by the cackle of kookaburras, and nocturnal fruit bats keep us

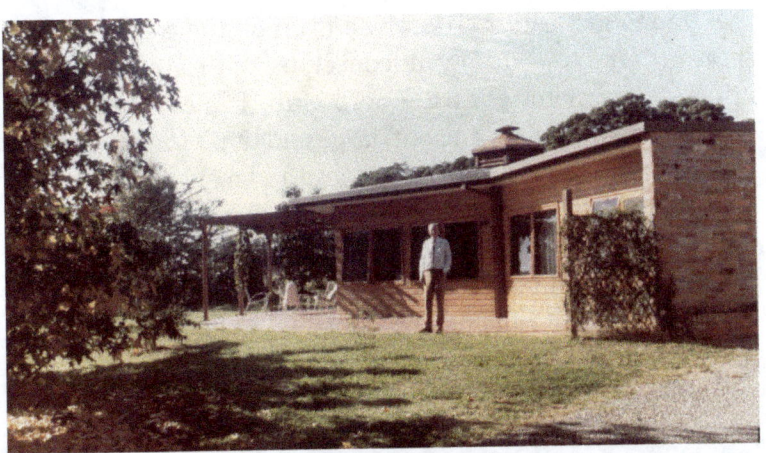

"Apuldram" in the North Boambee Valley, Coffs Harbour

from our beauty sleep when the mangos are ripening, but it is still a paradise.

During those years with Rainy Macdonald, we had our share of triumphs and disasters. Three separate head injuries illustrate the difficulties of being away from the city super-specialists. There was no air ambulance, and transfer meant an eight hour drive by road ambulance crossing some of the northern NSW rivers by ferry.

A semi-conscious Boy Scout arrived in the ambulance, having been hit on the back of his head by a stone which had been skipped on a river surface by his friends. He soon became deeply unconscious. Meanwhile I had contacted the Air Force as their planes were sometimes called on for emergency evacuation. During the next four hours, I was referred up the line of command, a difficult task as no-one would take responsibility for approval of this expensive exercise. It was also the late evening on a holiday weekend. His condition deteriorated and I was forced to undertake cerebral decompression, but he died just as the Air Force rang to say that they were preparing a plane.

A young girl had been hit by a train on the track near her caravan, and was deeply unconscious with an open brain injury. As a member of the aero club, I knew that an old Norseman aircraft, an ancient, large and lumbering high wing work horse was on the tarmac, doing aerial survey work with a magnetometer pulled behind it on a long cable. They agreed to take us to Brisbane, fortunately in good weather. During the ninety minute flight, I continually administered paralysing agents to stop her fitting and controlled her breathing with oxygen via an intra-tracheal tube. At the Brisbane hospital, I handed over gratefully to the neurosurgical staff but the patient's injuries were too severe for survival.

There I met an extraordinary man, neurosurgeon Ken Jamieson, who invited me to stay at his home overnight. We talked for hours and finally, I went to bed at 1 a.m., but Ken stayed up working till 2 a.m. and got up at 5 a.m. He stated he had a terrible family history of early deaths by heart attack and was determined to pack everything he could into his short life. When not operating or seeing patients, he was doing a survey of fatal and near-fatal road accidents, with a team of police, pathologists, psychologists and others whose expertise was relevant. Curiously, when Ken was depressed, he would not bother with a seat belt, although his studies showed clearly this increased safety factor. He did die young of his family curse, but not before saving the third case.

The teenage daughter of an aero club friend fell off her horse, hitting the back of her head on hard ground. An X-ray showed a linear fracture of the back of the skull. She was in a strange stuporose state, with very little to find on clinical examination, except an upgoing toe on stimulating the sole of the foot, the Babinski reflex. Normally, the toe curls downwards and this curious test is of very great importance. Ken had given me a slim book he had published for medical students and junior doctors, and this emphasised the danger of this sign, when increasing pressure at the back of the brain could cone the brain stem down, compressing it and its vital breathing and cardiac centres. The girl's father was prepared to fly in a specialist in a chartered plane. I phoned Ken, he had no immediate commitments and arrived at dusk, carrying a bundle of special instruments.

Within half an hour the theatre was prepared and she stopped breathing on her own just as Rainy intubated her lungs. Ken quickly decompressed the back of her brain, a very tricky area close to so many vital structures. We found blood had been seeping under pressure from the great veins across the fracture line. It was a very close call. She flew back with him on a stretcher in the same chartered plane and made a full recovery. I saw her the other day. She has no memory of that fortnight.

One evening, I was putting the first forkful of tea to my mouth when the phone rang. "My husband has just shot himself," said a quiet voice, so quiet I assumed it was a minor injury. "In his stomach," she continued. Tea was instantly forgotten as I raced up to the hospital. He had upended a gun to finish killing a snake with the butt and had left a bullet in the breach, as I had done ten years previously in Azare. Rainy bled eight donors from our panel whilst I put up a drip, cross-matched the blood and arranged for an immediate operation. We left the theatre six hours later, having removed his tattered spleen, sewn up the hole in his stomach and removed a segment of his gut. The bullet had finally lodged under the skin of his back, having also clipped a nerve to his leg. He had a totally uneventful recovery and died twenty years later from a heart attack. Jill reheated my supper, a piece of by now dried up fish and I finished it in peace at 2 a.m.

Tetanus is a great rarity in western countries, thanks to immunisation in childhood. Early in my partnership, I met a middle-aged patient who lived in the valley close to where we eventually settled. Nellie and her husband ran cattle and a banana plantation and she came to the surgery on many occasions with minor scratches and wounds, but had always refused to have either prophylactic or immunising tetanus injections.

"It's not natural," she said however much I pleaded with her. The final choice lies with the patient except for contagious cases like tuberculosis, but I obtained her signature on a piece of paper to that effect. Whenever she came to see me, we had a little joke,

"Got tetanus, have we?"

Twenty-five years later, her neighbour rang up to report Nellie was very unwell. As I walked into her room, I made our inevitable little joke. "I think it is, doctor," she replied as her back stiffened in spasm, and it was. She had begun to notice stiffness whilst hanging out the washing. I found a small wood splinter with a bead of pus in her seventy-five year old ankle, the ideal spot for the bacteria to flourish in oxygen free conditions, and to deliver its toxin to her nervous system. She was admitted and given anti-toxin and antibiotics, but once the poison has latched onto the nerve endings, it takes weeks to disappear. She was flown to Sydney and spent six weeks in St. Vincent's Hospital, kept paralysed and asleep on artificial respiration. She made a full recovery and went dancing again three months later.

I was discussing tetanus several years later with a new partner and mentioned her name.

"Nellie," he exclaimed, "I know Nellie very well." He had met his wife, an intensive care sister, and done much of his courting at Nellie's bedside when he was a junior doctor.

The work of a general practitioner is mostly a daylong grind, often with night calls for emergencies or maternity cases when the next day seems to go on for hours longer than normal. Tempers become frayed and have to be rigidly controlled. The patient is not interested in the fact that the doctor feels worse than he does. He has paid for an opinion and not a confrontation. After an irritated outburst, I have immediately felt so guilty that I have been extra effusive, to make up the psychologically correct degree of caring which I should have shown.

Every few months a tense clinical situation would arise, instantly recognised by Jill by my silence and restlessness at night. It could be due to unexpected post-operative surgical complications, a sick new-born baby or an antagonistic relative. Those few days were spent in anxiety, headache from lack of sleep and a decrease in efficiency. After the crisis had resolved, the weight lifted from my shoulders but had added another grey hair to my head.

I grew to recognise impending, unavoidable situations with a sinking feeling, knowing I faced more sleepless nights. This is an aspect of medicine that only doctors and their wives understand. Outwardly, we keep a brave, self-possessed and calm facade, but the preoccupation impairs our judgement with other patients. If you think your doctor looks quieter than usual, treat him or her kindly, they may be going through one of these difficult periods, and is a candidate for an early heart attack.

I savoured the many lighter moments. Our first Coffs Harbour friend Roy Riddel, an ex-Spitfire pilot dentist, sent his sixteen year old daughter in for a penicillin injection. She hitched up her skirt, pulled down the top of her pants to show a target Roy had painted on her hip with textacolour. "Dad says hit that," she announced. Roy had a habit of waiting until Jill was in his dental chair with her mouth open and her voice inoperative to discuss how he and I were going to buy an expensive plane together.

Nurse Hazel in the operating theatre, besides being a great nurse, was and is the source of the most constructive malapropisms, a malapropist of genius. I was given new white operating theatre boots which she remarked on.

"Virginal white," I said.

"Yes," she replied, "like the immaculate contraception."

Her favourite film star is Lawrence of Olivier and, on a tour in China, she asked if they had problems with rape and incense. Following an argument with the hierarchy, she was so angry, she was "rapeable", the Australian term being "ropeable".

We hosted many fourth or fifth year medical students who had to see general practice as an important and previously overlooked part of their medical education. As a student myself, based at a teaching hospital, I had had no idea of what it entailed as a separate discipline. The College of General Practice had been set up to delineate the functions of a GP and encourage its members. Certain practices were approved for student training for two week terms.

Most of our students wanted to stay longer. Their eyes had been opened to the wide range of cases seen. They realised that between the steady flow of coughs, arthritis and diarrhoea, were fascinating and often serious clinical problems to be dealt with promptly and efficiently. Most patients were co-operative in having young strangers sitting in, but we always gave them the opportunity to request privacy, suggesting the student take a coffee break. There was a wide variation in their abilities. Some, with only six months to go before qualifying, gave their first injections, pelvic examinations and ear washouts in our rooms, whilst others were extremely well prepared with a wealth of up to date knowledge which I gratefully absorbed.

At the age of 55, after 22 years of general practice, I found the constant night calls for maternity, anaesthetics and emergencies becoming very tiring. I applied for the post of hospital Medical Superintendent at the Coffs Harbour Hospital, which had just become vacant, little realising that it was not to be the more relaxed life style I had expected.

CHAPTER 16: HOSPITAL SUPERINTENDENT

My position as medical superintendent of Coffs Harbour Hospital had been extended to take in three outlying hospitals: Bellingen, Dorrigo and Macksville. I found I was on thirtyseven committees. The individual board meetings varied with the hospital's character. Coffs Harbour District Hospital was in the late adolescent stage, growing up to become a base hospital with a wide range of specialists and their technical requirements.

Bellingen board at the time was unsympathetic towards the medical staff who were treating the high proportion of alternative life-style patients with sympathy. The Macksville doctors were antagonistic towards their board, which they correctly felt was under instructions from the Health Department to decrease the range of procedures.

Dorrigo board had relaxed meetings seen through a haze of cigarette smoke emanating from the chairman who occasionally turned blue in a spasm of coughing. They were interested in the minor problems, as the hospital was being downgraded to take only long term nursing home cases or simple conditions. Even the maternity section was closed, as it was felt that twenty cases a year was insufficient to maintain expertise. A small amount of funding was made available to each hospital yearly for dentures, and the Dorrigo chairman would wheeze comments such as, "No, old Fred lives in a caravan near us. He seems to eat his steaks normally. I don't think he needs choppers."

My functions were to provide medical expertise to the boards on all administrative matters, and to liaise between the Health Department and the medical staff. Relations were always strained, as the philosophy of the doctors was to maintain their independence in all medical matters, whilst the department was trying to introduce some form of discipline in management and expenditure. Both sides were right. There should be only one captain of the ship for treatment, or chaos ensues, but some curb had to be placed on the extravagant use of drugs, equipment, pathology tests and radiology. The third corner of the therapeutic triangle was the patient with the relatives demanding the best of both worlds. Those who had previously neglected an elderly family member became aggressively vocal when they sensed the end was approaching, a latent guilty feeling perhaps. There is a tendency amongst some doctors to feel that death indicates failure and to order tests and treatment which would influence neither comfort nor outcome. I found one terminal lung cancer man had been given eighty bottles of intravenous fluids and twenty-six blood tests in the month of dying, when morphia alone would have been the kindest way of easing his passing.

A general practitioner, benignly caring for the welfare of patients, sits behind his desk saying, "I'm going to give you these tablets," not strictly accurate as the prescriptions are heavily subsidised by the Health Department. As medical superintendent, I was thrust into the harsh economic world of budgets and cutbacks, and resentment and indignation from staff and patients' relatives. It soon became apparent that either a short explanation of circumstances, or a few minutes listening would solve most problems, but I found it very hard to be the whipping boy for government policy or poor communication by doctors.

I conducted a survey of all the complaints for the previous two years and found most came from relatives, and nine out of ten were against doctors who had not been guilty of malpractice, but who had failed to take a few minutes to talk, some of them having what I labelled "Incipient Divinity".

The Health Department held a short seminar on "Stress and Burnout", and tried to teach us to relax by listening to soft music which I found a waste of time as I was already too well versed in Beethoven and Mozart to make my mind a blank page. However, a psychiatrist gave me the best advice. "What you have got to remember," he said, "is that the main function of a medical administrator is to absorb anger." I found it amusing that we should be given stress management courses by the department which itself was the main stressor. "The department giveth, the department taketh away, Blessed be the name of the department," I announced at one regional office conference. I notice now how everybody associated with an unpleasant occurrence is counselled but the medical and nursing staff never had nor requested this privilege. It was all part of medical life but might have saved the occasional suicide by younger doctors who took their patients' deaths as personal failures.

As Coffs Harbour Hospital was being built up to become a full base hospital, the easy-going habits of the older doctors had to be re-examined. No longer could anyone with a medical degree walk into the operating theatre and perform whatever he felt he was capable of doing. Likewise, certain serious medical conditions had to have a second opinion by a specialist, now that we had a wide range of these highly qualified persons.

"Delineation of privileges" became the watch words, which generated considerable antagonism, until it was pointed out that it would be phased in slowly and would still allow competent doctors to continue their practices under a "grandfather" clause. It was more for future generations, and would be carried out by a committee with a majority of doctors. The unpleasant alternative would have been a decree from the Health Department. The general practitioners were increasingly busy at their own rooms, and most surgery was passed over to the surgical specialists with some relief. The upsurge in technology in the medical field, cardiac monitoring and endoscopic examinations of the upper and lower gut and lungs needed specially trained physicians.

Conditions were laid down for calling in a gynaecologist for complications of pregnancy and childbirth, and certain childrens' diseases had to have a paediatric opinion. The divergence between general practitioners and specialists has been widened by the huge increase in procedural medical defence (malpractice) premiums, so that it needed thirty maternity cases to break even with the cost of such insurance, and occasional surgery would run at a loss. There were limits to the number of positions for specialist and general practitioner appointments based on population forecasts.

A medical establishment was set up, which was supposed to keep costs down, on the theory that any new doctor would use more bed space, pathology tests and radiology. This seemed to ignore the finite number of beds and patients in the Coffs Harbour district.

We were expected to start quality assurance programs, and I spent a few days in Sydney being indoctrinated into the process. First a potential problem had to be recognised, then surveyed by questionnaires. The results were tabulated when deficiencies would become recognisable. Efforts were then made to rectify these and the final part occurred at a specified date in the future when the results were to be reassessed. That was the theory.

I found that many doctors did not think there were any problems with their work, and no doubt felt threatened despite the assurance that there was no criticism. Some were worried lest any adverse results could be used in later malpractice cases. We therefore started with more domestic issues such as patient satisfaction and comfort. Questionnaires had to be carefully written with no double or leading questions. I spoke at a quality assurance conference about a hand injury survey we did in the accident department, "but no-one wrote back". The audience roared with laughter. If we found a problem, such as the hardness of the beds in intensive care ward, we made plans to rectify it. Finally, a definite date was made for review in six to twelve months. I could feel the increasing discipline of a major hospital in the making. The easygoing days were fading.

I revived the art of "shroud waving", which had been used on me as a GP many times by patients wanting instant treatment. "Better come straight away, doc. It could be a coroner's case," would always induce an urgent visit, even though I knew from past experience that I would find a patient with a simple cold and certainly not moribund. Some specialists attempted to use the technique on me, to obtain more up-to-date equipment, which I had to balance against the budget and the other specialist's requests.

"I won't be responsible if a child dies," was passed on to regional office with alacrity and sometimes cynicism. We set up an equipment committee of assorted specialists and nursing staff, and "prioritised" a list of their requests, to use the jargon of the administration. I personally invented a new verb which I presented to a regional conference and dedicated to the deputy director, an efficient young woman trained in social work. "We have to pragmatise," I announced to great applause from the gathered medical superintendents, chief executive officers and directors of nursing.

It had taken twenty-five years to build the present hospital and looked like taking equally as long for extensions which were now desperately needed. The first plan envisaged building an extra ward and a new ten bedded intensive care ward on top of the main ward, with an enlarged operating theatre, X-ray unit, pathology and pharmacy. The administration block was to be shifted to separate new buildings to make way for the new casualty department. After a year or so of consideration, discussions and interdepartmental committees, the whole plan was scrapped as being too disruptive to the other wards whilst under construction.

A second plan was then drawn up by a firm of architects for a huge extension doubling its size. This took another two years and was scrapped as being too grandiose and expensive. A third plan on a less ambitious scale allowing a space for later beds under its extended wing was presented by the Health Department.

Meanwhile a "green fields" total rebuild on neighbouring flat ground had been mentioned and dismissed. The third plan was scrapped and it was decided to use the original plan, emptying the underlying ward during the noisiest part of the construction into less essential rooms around the hospital.

The casualty front office became a very uncomfortable intensive care ward and a temporary series of offices (which looked suspiciously permanent) housed the exploding administrative population. Fifteen years later, in 2001, a totally new complex was built on the green fields site, so all the million or more dollars of taxpayers' money for the other shelved plans had been wasted.

In response to many requests, we decided to build a hospital chapel, which was done within one year paid for by public contributions. I met the ministers fraternal (or "For Eternal" as Sheila, my secretary, so creatively mistyped) and decided on the layout which would fit an extension on a concrete cantilever platform outside the surgical ward entrance. From then on, I dispensed with committees. Sheila and I coordinated the fund raising and building, which came in exactly on budget, a far cry from the squandering of public money for the three hospital plans. A local artist designed a set of three stained glass windows in an ecumenical style so that it could be used by any religious denomination, Christian, Jewish, Moslem or Sikh. They represented the sea and its bounty, the local agriculture and the forests and mountains, with a dove, the international symbol of peace, overhead. It was regularly used by those in need of spiritual comfort, and as an overnight waiting room for anxious relatives. It now graces the pre-anaesthetic waiting room outside the 2001 hospital operating theatres.

The Regional Medical Director asked me to set up a cancer care unit, similar to the one he was setting up at Lismore. His own wife had to go to Sydney for treatment and the long journey took its toll on such very sick, debilitated patients, adding to their misery. An old house opposite the casualty entrance was for sale, and John Slater, the hospital secretary found a cache of funds for the purpose of land purchase. The oncology department of the Royal North Shore Hospital agreed to send specialists up by air on a regular basis for consultations and chemotherapy under the supervision of a trained nursing sister. Since its inception, it has grown from the original thirty patients to many hundreds, and now has sophisticated equipment, including a radiotherapy and chemotherapy wing in the 2001 hospital run by its own oncology specialists.

I had taken up the position, thinking that it would be less stressful than the continual night calls of general practice, midwifery and anaesthetics. The stress continued for unexpected reasons. Firstly, I had to give evidence against some colleagues which went completely against my ethics of supporting fellow doctors as prescribed in the Hippocratic oath. Torn between this and my duty to tell the truth in the witness box, in which I spent three and a half days, I developed a duodenal ulcer which took time to settle. I felt the matter should have been resolved amicably by the Health Department out of court, and it was not the best way to make friends and influence the medical staff in my new position. Indeed, most of my future dealings with that medical group was met with antagonism. The case was dropped, which was the correct result, but severely distressed all concerned.

Secondly, it was reported to me that five babies had been born with cleft palates within a few weeks of each other, with a sixth one previously that year. Statistically, the yearly average should have been two. I reported this to the regional office and an investigation was set in progress. All infant abnormalities, normally 5% per annum both major and minor, were audited.

We prepared a series of questions: both parent's backgrounds, work place, hereditary factors, diet, medications and exposure to chemicals, and compared them each with two families with normal babies born within the same weeks. The only tenuous correlation for all abnormalities was possibly the use of home pesticides. I suggested to a reporter that pregnant mothers should use a fly swat rather than a spray, and was awarded a newspaper headline, "Swat

Don't Spray", and a visit from the anxious managers of a Sydney spray can factory.

An anti-chemical group calling themselves "Women for Health" took part in meetings and debates and focussed on the banana crop-spraying aircraft, despite the fact that most of the cleft palates were well outside the area of drift at the time when the embryonic mouths were forming. Attempts to refute such accusations brought forth the cry of "cover-up", my definition of which is: "my preconceived ideas have not been confirmed by your scientific findings and you must therefore be hiding something".

The fact was not considered that we had nothing to hide and could have made a medical breakthrough. It was impossible to draw any statistical conclusions from such a small sampling as six cases, and over a span of several years, the figures showed that Coffs Harbour had the national average of all common abnormalities. However, the department demonstrated that it was prepared to investigate any potential problems, and it was a good exercise in quality control.

The media had a field day. The scenario had everything for both newspapers and television. There were mothers and babies to zoom cameras on to, villains in the shape of nasty, buzzy, lowflying crop-dusters, and a group of heroic ladies confronting the chemical industry, whilst the health professionals were obviously holding important facts back. Despite multiple totally normal tests, the purity of the drinking water was questioned. A Melbourne newspaper headlined "Paradise Lost", and even a doctor whose wife was in early pregnancy telephoned to ask me if it was safe to holiday in our dangerous atmosphere. It was a classical example of a media beat-up on the flimsiest of evidence and diminished my opinion of that profession.

Thirdly, an edict from the Health Minister which would have halved the income of most doctors caused a massive reaction from the profession. The high-handed statements that doctors who did not conform would be liable to lose their Medicare based income completely, started a withdrawal of services at all public hospitals for all except emergency cases or for those in pain. The interpretation of the patient status varied according to the medico-political views of individual doctors, and as the weeks progressed, more and more cases were declared as semi-emergencies.

I was asked by a sweet-talking female reporter what it was all about and I stated, "what else can they now do?" This was headlined the next day as "Hospital Chief Backs Strike," despite the fact that I was doing my best to keep the medical services running as efficiently as possible. I received an official rebuke from the department, but was told not to take it to heart as they knew the inaccuracies of the press only too well. From then on, I quoted Rudyard Kipling (who was himself a reporter) in his poem: *If*, to gentlemen and ladies of the media.

If you can bear to hear the truth you've spoken,

Twisted by knaves to set a trap for fools.

After several months, the minister withdrew his decrees, and left a medical profession no longer a loose association of doctors, quietly doing their own jobs in their own unobtrusive way, but a very powerful well organised group. The waiting lists had increased, as had medical suspiciousness. Militant politicisation had set in.

Lastly, this was the time of funding cuts. I went to numerous meetings in Lismore, the regional centre, which used the half empty Coraki Hospital as a conference centre. There, we discussed problems and solutions common to all areas. We felt sorry for the senior hierarchy who had been told to come in on budget despite the rapidly expanding population and diminishing funding. I vividly recall one hard mouthed Treasury official saying, "You will ignore the demands of the doctors, the patients and the general public. You will come in on budget." Contracts for the chief executive officers were for a fixed term of seven years with dismissal if the budget was exceeded, hardly conducive to entering the administrative service as a career.

The hospital was partly closed for Christmas, and there were six weeks of emergency admissions only, the declaration of which depended on the doctor, for no lay person would dare suggest that the condition could have waited another month.

"Shroud waving" reached new heights. "Are you going to be responsible if this patient dies?" I was the only administrator who could give a medical opinion. As I was older than any of the consultants, they respected my views, and generally kept within the restrictions, whilst I would never turn down requests for admission which were obviously necessary for the patient's welfare. I did not like playing God under these circumstances. The administration enjoyed Christmas as a time of reduced expenditure and the staff as a time of relative quietness.

One Christmas Eve was not so quiet. In the casualty department balloons and coloured trimmings festooned the walls, wishing an unlikely Merry Christmas to those unfortunate enough to have need of our attention. The staff flaunted Santa Claus badges on their uniforms and spoiled their appetites with excessive snacks of nuts, chocolates and junk food, but avoided the side tables laden with bottles of beer, wine and spirits, at least until their duty time finished. The operating theatres were closed except for emergencies.

We did not expect any activity until after Christmas Day, when the annual Sydney surf-seekers arrived in their thousands to outnumber us, expecting City facilities which we strived to deliver with our scant resources.

Mid-morning, the ambulance rang to tell us to expect a desperately ill nine month old infant of alternative lifestyle parents from the Kalang valley in the Bellingen area. The local doctors had given him immediate and appropriate penicillin for suspected meningitis. On arrival in casualty, he was found to be in extremis with a fulminating infection and the typical meningitis rash. He died within ten minutes. The distraught parents told us that a few days before they had attended the Christmas gathering of between two and four hundred similar lifestyle people from a wide area of the northern NSW coast. Their extended family spirit ensured that everyone shared each others' company and food, and babies were handed around, admired, and sometimes mutually breast-fed. It was a potential epidemic and needed urgent action.

It was just before closing time at the head office at Lismore, when I rang for information and help. The high background noise of music, laughter and chinking glasses indicated that the staff had decided that their duty time had finished. The public health officials had left early, and the remaining upper hierarchy seemed uncertain of procedures and showed a certain unwillingness to become too involved at a distance of one hundred and fifty kilometres.

"Carry on, Jelliffe, I'm sure you can cope. Take as many throat swabs as possible and give prophylactic antibiotics to everyone who had been in contact. Merry Christmas."

The best prophylactic antibiotic was Rifampicin which is used mainly in the treatment of tuberculosis. Coffs Harbour had a very small supply and we contacted Grafton Hospital, which was the TB treatment centre, eighty kilometres north. The police had skeleton staffs at both towns, but arranged for a car to deliver the drug, meeting a Coffs Harbour car midway. The only other prophylaxis was old fashioned sulphadiazine, which neither the hospital nor the chemists stocked any more, except as a veterinary product, and was ineffective for some strains of meningitis. We had to rely on the Rifampicin.

The main problem was to reach the possible contacts, most of whom had departed home to other communities many kilometres away, or in the shady recesses of the Kalang valley. The Bellingen Health Inspector arranged to hold an immediate clinic in the valley's community hall, for distribution of Rifampicin, and to take throat swabs. Few residents had telephones and the information was passed around by word of mouth. About one hundred and fifty turned up, and fortunately, there were no positive swabs and no further cases.

The Health Inspector and I decided to approach the Kalang valley residents to assess our performance, and make adequate contingency plans. I met with a committee of five, four being keen to help, but one woman was very reserved and suspicious of our motives. After a while, she realised that we were completely non-judgemental and had no intention of interfering with her chosen lifestyle, and she then co-operated enthusiastically.

The devastating sudden death had lead many residents to accept standard medicine, and we offered to send out public health and immunisation pamphlets. The main problem as we all saw it was the difficulty in communication in a scattered community. We had not used the local radio station until late, forgetting its potential. The resident committee decided to set up a communication network. We parted with mutual respect and a plan for dealing with any future disastrous situations. It was a Christmas to remember.

An infectious disease in a bus can pose problems. A year later, a bus load of Boy Scouts called in at Coffs Harbour, with one early case of meningitis. Throat swabs were taken from thirty reluctant little boys, gagging vigorously, some saying they were unable to swallow tablets. A worse public health risk was a local school bus driver with a cough, who had open tuberculosis. A large number of students had to have X-rays and Mantoux skin tests, with follow up for months.

There were bright spots, too. On a late December day, an eighteen month old girl was rushed into casualty by her mother who was a nurse. Laura was unconscious with dilated pupils, blue, wheezing and frothing from the lungs, with a pulse rate of two hundred. The anaesthetist intubated her in the operating theatre to ensure her oxygen supply, and the paediatrician did a lumbar puncture to exclude meningitis. Her family had come from Western Australia to visit relatives at Coramba, in the hills 15 km from Coffs Harbour and she had been having a sleep on a mattress on the floor in the overcrowded house. Despite the lack of any marks, the symptoms fitted funnel web spider bite, which gives an effect like a huge dose of adrenaline. We had recently received a small supply of the experimental antivenene made from rabbit serum, the only animal which can produce sufficient amounts. The child was dying so there was nothing to lose. We followed the protocol and slowly injected two ampoules. Within ten minutes, the chest had cleared, her pulse was normal and she awoke with nothing worse than a sore throat and a bad temper from the sedatives.

The spider bite was found hidden under the shoulder. Her mother sent me Laura's photograph next year and assured me she did not have any after effects, and knowing the antidote came from rabbits, was not unduly interested in carrots. Fourteen years later, I presented Laura's case to a medical meeting on envenomation, and Laura's mother sent me a photograph of Laura in evening dress for her school ball. It lifted my spirits tremendously.

A fifteen year old boy had ignored the traffic lights and had been knocked off his bicycle, suffering a severe head injury. He was deeply unconscious and was on a life support system, lungs inflated with oxygen from a mechanical respirator. He was brain dead, which we verified by the five criteria laid down by the organ transplant ethics committee. As he had no hope of recovery, we discussed the possibility of his becoming an organ donor, a first for Coffs Harbour, and contacted the organ transplant unit in Sydney, who agreed to take him if the relatives agreed.

Interviewing the family was one of the most distressing tasks I have ever undertaken, as bad as telling people they are dying. They were still trying to come to terms with the loss of a strongly built young son, and found it difficult to accept that he was technically dead. His heart, lungs, liver and kidneys had to be removed from his seemingly live body, as they were of no use once the life support system was closed down. The most difficult member to convince was his grandmother, and it required all my tact and persuasion to convince her to let her beloved grandson go. Finally, they gave permission, and certification by three independent doctors confirmed that he was legally suitable for organ donation.

From a distance of six hundred kilometres this required meticulous timing. The organs have only a short life span outside the body, even when cooled to near freezing. There were to be five recipients who had to be checked for compatibility and prepared for immediate surgery. Often, they had been waiting at home for this call for weeks or months.

As evening approached, wild storm clouds built up as a cold front swept up the coast. The first team to harvest the kidneys and liver arrived, pale after a rough ride in a small twin engined aircraft dodging the storm cells. It appeared over the aerodrome in a Wagnerian manner in keeping with the death and transfiguration scenario about to be performed. A flash of lightning struck the hospital, putting its all important telephone line out of action. The pay phone in the foyer remained serviceable and the nursing Sister used her plastic phone card to keep the Sydney hospitals informed of progress.

As the first team finished its work, a twin engined Lear jet loaned for such occasions by its media magnate owner, landed and the cardiac team arrived, fresh from their flight above the turbulent weather. Within thirty minutes, they were back in the air, to be taken across Sydney by fast ambulance. By an extraordinary coincidence, the heart recipient was a Coffs Harbour man, who had the most compatible tissue and blood type.

The family dispersed sadly, with the consolation that five people could now live normal lives. It seemed to comfort them a little in their nightmare. For the next few days, I had a series of unpleasant dreams, in which I had removed all the abdominal organs from a normal person and had to apologise to the relatives waiting outside.

Another stormy night, we had more drama when a twinengined commuter aircraft missed the runway and plowed into the low coastal bushes between the airfield and the beach. We had annual dress rehearsals for such emergencies, but in daylight, in readily accessible sites. The real thing was totally different. The control tower could see the fire but was unsure of its exact position for ambulance access. One of our psychiatric nurses flew a helicopter and quickly located it with its searchlight, and started to evacuate some of the burnt passengers, landing very dramatically in the hospital car park. The ambulance itself had some difficulty in getting to the site in thick scrubland. Two passengers and the pilot were dead, and the other major injuries were burns.

At a later debriefing, the ambulance staff queried the helicopter's incursion into their operations. This was not surprising as it was not included in the previous exercises, but nevertheless I felt it proved its worth in the special circumstances. One criticism was that there was no counselling of victims and relatives, until it was pointed out that the counsellor himself was an injured passenger. The accident highlighted the differences between a pleasant, daytime, fair weather, easily accessible exercise in good visibility and the real thing.

This was the time of the boat people escaping from South Vietnam where the communists had taken over, and anyone with capitalist activities was under suspicion or persecuted. Most of them were ethnic Chinese and were living in our cities, until they could be found employment. Some local church groups decided to help in a practical way, and approached us to use our open plan cottage next to our house, as temporary accommodation.

They assumed quite incorrectly that these people would be proficient gardeners. We assumed we would be taking one family, but were asked to have two: four adults and six children. When we raised our eyebrows and suggested that congestion would occur, it was pointed out that in the Indonesian and other transit camps, they were crowded together as thickly as the bananas in our plantation.

Two delightful families came, the children ranging from a fourteen year old girl to a very new baby. The men went out to work getting housing and an agricultural plot ready, but they were city folk, having previously worked in an import-export business and as foreman in a textile mill. Their knowledge of gardening was minimal, but their enthusiasm to help was maximal.

I had my sit-on mower commandeered and numerous small plants accidentally run over. Every Saturday, appetising aromas wafted out of their house and Thanh, the daughter, would appear with a bowl of delicious soup, in which floated various unidentifiable objects which we never recognised. Jill tried to teach the mothers a little English, but the children rapidly became fluent in school. After five months, they decided to return to friends in Sydney, where the men took on two jobs each and no doubt the children will have worked hard and had good educations, like most of the highly motivated migrants.

In February 1987, I suddenly felt hemmed in and irritated, and needed a change. I booked two seats to Wellington in New Zealand two weeks ahead. Jill spluttered that she had too many engagements, but came all the same. We had a wonderful time driving to Te Anau, walking up steep trails and seeing Milford Sound. Jill felt tired and when we arrived back, she discovered a lump in her remaining breast. Peter Gerard performed a mastectomy, and she went to Sydney for a six week course of radiotherapy, although the pathology report gave a favourable outlook. Twenty-two years later, she remains well.

By 1988, I had begun to feel my work as administrator irksome, and cut off from my fellow doctors. My sixtieth birthday came up enabling me to resign and claim my superannuation savings. My old partners agreed to have me back part-time, without midwifery or anaesthetics, and I found myself upstairs next to my previous consulting room, happily back with real medicine. I took me three days to retrieve my old medical patter and to catch up with advances in treatment, as I had attended most of the lectures and seminars available during my five years as medical superintendent. I have not taken part in any further hospital politics. "There's nothing so ex as an ex."

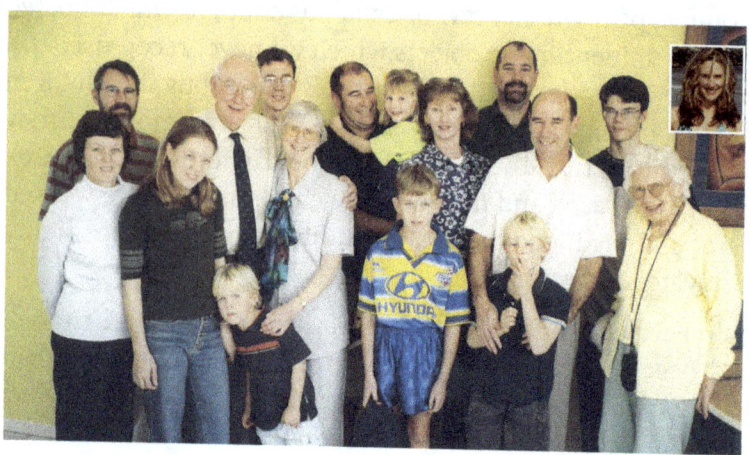

50th wedding anniversary, 2nd June 2001.
From left: Kathy & Michael, Kylie, William, Robin, Timothy, Jill, John holding Jessica, James, Evelyn, Rick, Peter with Jack, Cameron and Auntie Joan
Insert: Lisa

CHAPTER 17: FINAL STRETCH

I finally retired from general practice in 2004. I have now passed that rather daunting and mystic barrier of four score years. There was no sudden deterioration in my health or mental state, just the inexorable onset of irritating minor complaints, the sort I used to brush off as inconsequential in my elderly patients twenty or thirty years ago.

I can now identify with these old friends who made up most of my practice, with incurable but manageable conditions.

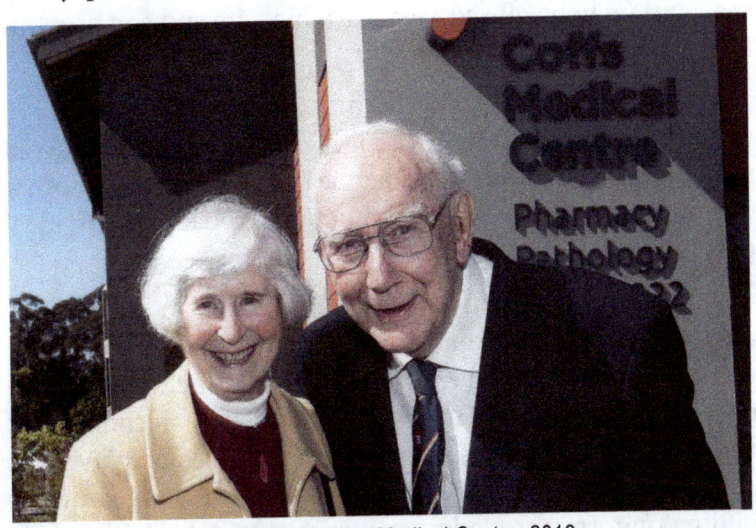

Opening of the new Medical Centre, 2013

The readily treatable, instant-cure younger patients see the younger doctors. I peered through trifocal lenses at skin lesions. I pushed my stethoscope more firmly into my ears to catch fading heart sounds. I double checked the correct doses of the plethora of present day potent medications. But I still got moments of extreme personal satisfaction, when I identified an early and treatable meningitis, an unusual and operable pancreatic tumour or an impending heart attack. And I am amused by the efforts of much younger social workers to push the elderly into physical routines which they do not want and physically cannot do. Just wait till they reach seventy plus years of age!

Jill and I had been visiting my old retired partner Rainy at the private hospital where he was being nursed for a terminal condition. He had been dozing peacefully, when he looked up, said, "I feel crook," and closed his eyes. I had been holding his hand at the time and felt his pulse stop. "Ask Sister for a stethoscope," I said to Jill, and confirmed that he had indeed slipped away, quietly without fuss, like the gentleman he always was, with his wife and son present. It was a deeply moving moment.

We had been partners for so many years without an angry word between us. We had both leant over backwards to avoid possible confrontations, and had learnt to rely on each other during many anxious medical moments. It had been an ideal partnership.

Twice weekly, I still assist the surgeons in the private operating theatres, keeping up my surgical interest without the responsibilities and anxieties of a sometimes stormy post-operative period. It is different in both technological and inter-personal ways from my student days of sixty years ago. Assisting at abdominal procedures no longer means pulling on retractor blades against taut muscles with aching arms, without the aid of muscle relaxants. The surgeon used to complain to the anaesthetist about the tight abdomen and the anaesthetist tried to keep the patient as deep as possible without killing them.

"If the patient can stay awake, surely you can, doctor," was countered by, "you realise if he gets any deeper, you will be conducting a post-mortem."

Sixty years ago, the nursing staff stood back in respectful reverence as the surgeon strode in masterfully to scrub and gown up. Loud whispering was suppressed by a sweeping glance from theatre Sister's gimlet eyes. Temper tantrums were acceptable behaviour for a great man under stress. Present day nursing staff are often highly qualified and respected not just as doctors' assistants, but as having heavy responsibilities of their own. The theatre atmosphere is more relaxed with soft taped music playing behind the anaesthetic trolley, and the murmur of conversation is accepted, except during tense moments, when Sister will request silence.

The extraordinary expansion of medical technology has allowed us to make accurate diagnoses through pathology tests and medical imaging, even in three dimensions. Laparoscopic surgery through tiny abdominal incisions using telescopic video cameras has replaced the incisions "big enough to put your head in". Fibre-optic light flowing from bright light sources have replaced the tiny light bulbs in the end of instruments, which failed when the electric current was turned up sufficiently to see with any degree of clarity.

Unlike the surgeon, the assistant often has time to let his mind wander. At the beginning and end of every procedure, a chorus of nurses' voices count the number of swabs, forceps and needles, to protect the patient, the surgeon's reputation and medical defence union. I have heard this so many times in so many accents, it is like a well-loved piece of music. I imagine a Mexican Wave of soft tones spreading round and round the countries of the world, following the sunrise and the opening of sterile packets of instruments. "One, two, three" in the varying dialects of the British Isles, followed by the twang of America.

"Hitotsu, futatsu, mittsu" from Japan, "Yi, er, san" from China are pursued by Russian and numerous European tongues, "Eins, zwei, drei" and "Un, deux, trois", not forgetting our old friends of Nigerian days, "Daya, biyu, uku". The discipline of the world's operating theatres has no ethnic boundaries.

For five years, I worked part-time for the Australian Government Health Service, assessing clients (the politically correct term for patients) with medical problems for eligibility for a disability pension. The sequence of events started with a statement from a local doctor, often appallingly written and just a diagnosis without confirmatory pathology, radiological or specialist's reports. I regarded these with suspicion, as no doctor is going to risk losing a patient from his practice by stating on a form which the client is going to read, that a pension is not needed.

A government-appointed doctor then formally takes a history and examines the relevant parts. He may also have to obtain the missing reports, often by fax machine. The senior medical officer then assesses all the evidence and gives a rating from a booklet with twenty-seven sections, from effort intolerance for heart and lungs, through limbs, spine, psychiatric to gynaecological, and that most useful part, miscellaneous.

Many applicants were genuine, but there was a hard core of socio-economic problems which were not medical and would be fit for useful light work.

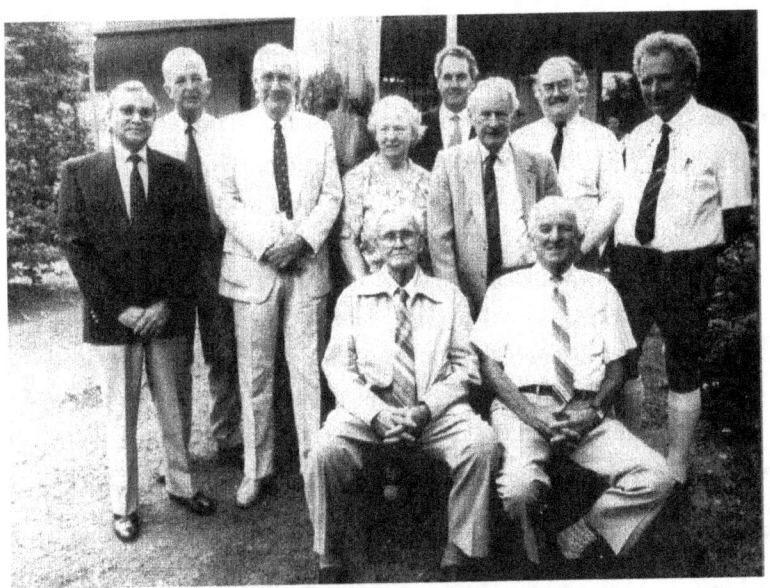

Visiting doctors at Baringa Hospital, 1993.
Dr. Rainy Macdonald seated in front left.

"But who will employ a fifty-year old man with back ache, when workers' compensation premiums will be excessive and no employer will take me?"

At the other end of the scale are the alcoholics and drug users, who candidly state they will take as much as they can afford. A pension enables them to keep their habits going and eventually contributes to their early demise. This ethical problem has been avoided by the authorities. However, my job was to give an opinion on medical matters, not ethics, and I adhered to the book in a non-judgemental manner.

There was a lighter side to this otherwise humourless activity, in the shape of some creative spelling mistakes and statements from both clients and doctors. One woman reported she suffered from the "manopause." Another had an "anginogram." And one had worked at a sewing machine all her life, and it would "seam" her muscles had worn out.

One man was late for an interview with a psychologist for poor memory, as he forgot.

Someone who had had two years "constricted" service had a "schizofreak" episode. "Knombeness" of the hands and feet, "eyeritis", "deepression", "condromalaysia", "whipelash" injury, "austroarthritis", "migrant" attacks, "mini-ears" disease, "quarterzone" injections, "enclosing spondylitis" and spurs on the "verty-bare" are examples of people who cannot spell "properle". There was even a letter supposedly from a Dr. Fracs, which is the surgical degree FRACS.

I retired from my general practice aged 76, four years ago and since then, I have kept up with medicine in a gentler manner. In place of workers' compensation and pension medical examinations, I now see about five non-Australians weekly, who need their immigration visas renewed or initiated, the majority being healthy and young. There are occasional elderly relatives moving to live out their lives with their children in Australia. They have chest X-rays taken as well as the HIV blood test and general basic medical assessment and very rarely have any sinister medical conditions. I enjoy these multinational meetings, and can usually calm their anxieties about being unable to stay in Australia, although the final answer lies with the Immigration Department.

I am gradually decreasing my time as assistant in the operating theatre in the private hospital to allow the younger generation more practice. I also have the feeling that as an octogenarian, the younger generation regard me as slowing up, and they are right. I certainly used to think that way about those ancient mariners when I was a student or junior doctor. I also sign cremation forms for the local funeral directors, because legally two separate doctors must certify that a cremation is not hiding anything sinister. The newly

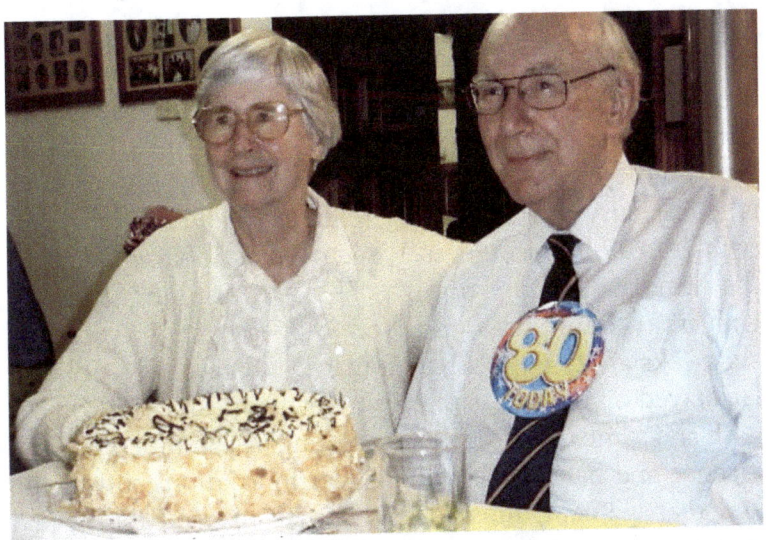

qualified hospital doctors frequently fill in death certificates incorrectly and time is spent in interviewing them to ensure the legality of my second certification. It also checks that any pacemaker or other implanted electrical apparatus has been removed, which would cause an explosion in the furnace.

But my great joy nowadays is to teach medical students. The old brick hospital building, built in 1970, was replaced in 2001 by a modern state-of-the-art hospital. A brand new medical school building was erected three years later, to take in 4th, 5th and 6th year medical students, as part of the University of New South Wales Rural School network, with other country towns, to ensure the availability of medical staff for the growing country population. There are several lecturers, some part-time like myself, and several local specialists and general practitioners. The students are impressive in their technical knowledge, and I attempt to teach them how to talk to, and examine living patients, who usually enjoy helping educate the future doctors.

I have had a lot of pleasure and sadness watching my four sons develop their interests in many unexpected ways. As a teenager, Michael, our eldest, became friendly with a dairy farmer in the Orara valley ten miles out of Coffs Harbour. He would cycle out every weekend and became an expert in practical dairy and pig farming, telling us about the delightful twinkle in their porcine eyes. We sent him to a boarding school, the Armidale School, known as TAS, and later, after a year at University, he went to visit New Guinea in 1971, spending six weeks assisting construction at Dauli Teacher's College. He stayed on in PNG gaining employment as a traffic officer with an airline there before completing his Commercial Pilot Licence and having a lifelong career in aviation, both flying and management, mostly in PNG. He married Kathy, and they have a primary school teacher daughter, Kylie, and two sons, Tim, and aeronautical engineer and computer database administrator, and Cameron, a primary school teacher.

We had the extreme sadness of losing our second son Peter, aged 49, in 2003 to a totally unexpected brain aneurysm whilst on holidays on the Barrier Reef. Peter had been an evironmental engineer with triple degrees, and at the forefront of his profession specialising in water. He was also an excellent guitarist and musician as well as sailor, having built a 40' ferro cement yacht. His daughter Lisa has a degree in visual communications working with advertising agencies in London, and has two younger sons, Jack and William.

He had been otherwise physically fit, and being confirmed as brain-dead by CT scan in Cairns hospital, he was offered for organ donation. We all agreed that Peter would have wished this and, indeed, he had been discussing this with his cousin, Christopher, who is an anaesthetist in Queensland, only one week before. The organ transplant unit initially kept us informed yearly about the recipients' progress. The heart man "has never stopped talking", one kidney and the liver were successful, but the other kidney and lungs did not last long. It made me appreciate how those other donors' families were strong enough to cope. In recognition of Peter's love of sailing, we held a short remembrance ceremony at the Coffs Harbour jetty after his funeral service, sliding his ashes into his favourite spot.

Our third son John is a sportsman, and is both a sailor and builder of boats and sailmaker. He learnt to fly and works as an air traffic controller at Brisbane. He lives on a large lychee farm to the north of Brisbane, and is married to Evelyn, who is a senior officer in the Queensland government's finance department. They have a tall athletic son, James and a mercurial daughter, Jessica.

Rick is our youngest son, who has gone into electronics and computers. He is a computer programmer who helped design some of the more advanced information technology languages and is the international Australian Standards committee representative in his field. It is all above my head, but I am proud of his achievements, as I am of all our sons'.

Computers, the internet and compact disc recording have arrived within the last twenty years. We have an array of such equipment, with a pile of ancient Bakelite records hiding sadly under the record player. I can take instant photographs with my digital camera, without worrying about the cost of film. The television is crystal clear, with multiple channels and the ability to record programs for later use. I can refer to anything, even medical problems, through the Google search engine.

I have watched enormous changes during my sixty clinical years, not only in treatment, but in demands for treatment, often triggered by exaggerated press reports. Alternative flavour of the month medicine comes and goes, often based on belief but not evidence. The greatest medical advance of the 1960s was the double blind trial. It is impossible to fudge results to confirm preconceived ideas, as the persons giving the treatment and collecting the results have no idea of what has been given or to whom. Evidence-based had become the watchword.

The market is constantly flooded with new medications, and the pharmaceutical reference book is expanding exponentially. The government has a constant headache trying to balance costs against efficacy, while the general public demands the best and the doctor is the meat in the sandwich. Many campaigns have been highly successful, such as the two-yearly Pap smear, and mammography, but occasionally, severe and even lethal drug side effects of a new medication have caused their withdrawal from the pharmacist's shelf. Patients are now requesting routine bone scans for osteoporosis, which makes sense in the long run, but cuts into the overstretched health dollar.

If I had been born a hundred years earlier, I would not have survived which was shown very clearly in the last three months, when I, at eighty, became a very sick, but now fully recovered patient. I recently had a very successful double cataract operation, with non-irritating plastic lenses inserted, going home within a few hours, a superb result. Totally unconnected was an upper abdominal pain two days later, which turned out to be an acutely inflamed gall-bladder, needing twice daily intravenous antibiotics, specialised X-rays and keyhole surgery resulting in bile leakage which needed a drain for a week. After carrying around a transparent hand-bag full of black drainage fluid, I had a visit to Port Macquarie hospital to see a specialist in the biliary tract. Under very light anaesthetic, he looked down my oesophagus and passed a fine drainage tube or stent to bridge the leaking hepatic duct, with instant complete relief.

I look back at all those lives which were wasted in my own family for lack of simple medical treatment which is taken for granted nowadays. The three uncles I never had, stillborn for want of a forceps or Caesarian delivery must have been a commonplace experience at the end of the 19th century. I look at the photograph of my sweet little blond would-have-been Aunt Winnie whose life could have been saved by an appendicectomy which today often keeps a patient in hospital for only one day.

How Grannie and Major Hebb must have felt their lives torn apart. And my own mother who should have had earlier breast cancer treatment and survived to enjoy a long life, like my own Jill. And patients like Leonora.

I have been very lucky to have lived in this time-slot. "May you live at an interesting time in history" is supposed to be a Chinese insult, but not in my case. I have been lucky in my father, my wife, my family, my work, my colleagues and my environment. I hope my last few years will be the same.

Apuldram

North Boambee Valley

2008

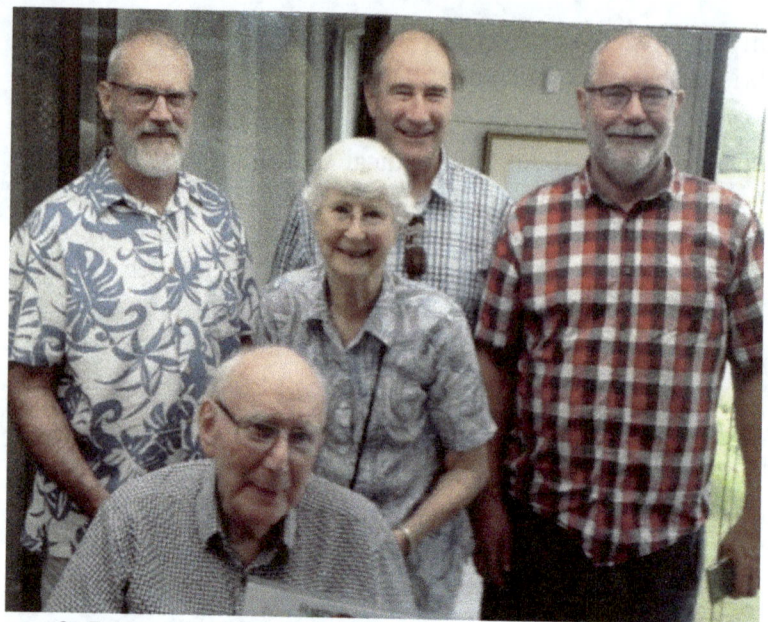

On Robin's 90th Birthday with Jill and (L-R) Michael, John & Rick, 2018

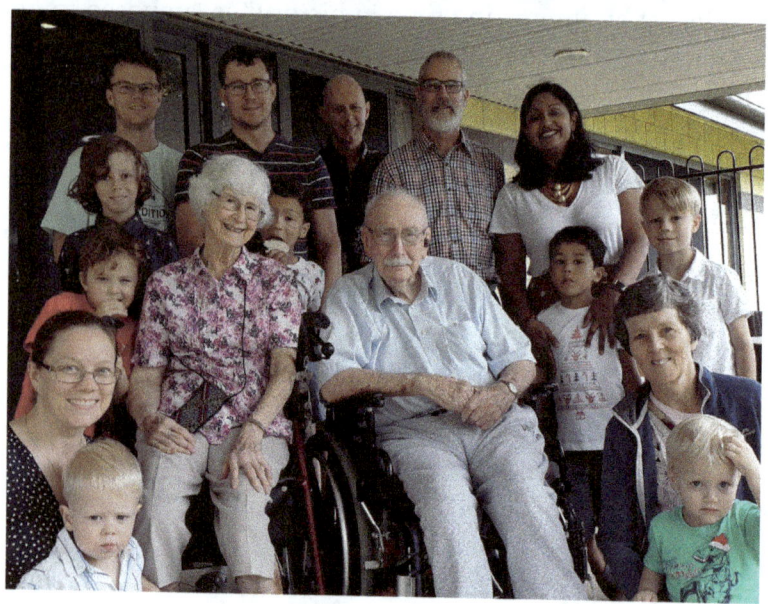

Robin & Jill with Michael & Kathy's family, Christmas 2019,
3 grandchildren, 7 great-grandchildren

Endnotes

1. With Robin's encouragement, Jill began to write her own story, later published in 2017, titled *I was Thursday's Child,* ISBN 978-0-6480675-1-1, available from Nenge Books (www.nengebooks.com) or through bookshops (print on demand).

2. The Territory of Papua and New Guinea (TPNG) was administerd by the Australian government until it achieved self-government in 1973, and Independence in Sept 1975, becoming Papua New Guinea.

3. Doug Parrington's story is recorded in his autobiography, *An Ongoing Journey - from Christian Work to Servanthood*, published by Nenge Books, ISBN 978-0-6480675-9-7, available from the publisher or bookshops (print on demand).

www.ingramcontent.com/pod-product-compliance
Lightning Source LLC
Chambersburg PA
CBHW050307010526
44107CB00055B/2137